CANCER TREATMENT

CHEMOTHERAPY AND RADIATION THERAPY

CANCER ETIOLOGY, DIAGNOSIS AND TREATMENTS

Additional books in this series can be found on Nova's website under the Series tab.

Additional e-books in this series can be found on Nova's website under the e-book tab.

CANCER ETIOLOGY, DIAGNOSIS AND TREATMENTS

CANCER TREATMENT

CHEMOTHERAPY AND RADIATION THERAPY

ANNE E. WILT
EDITOR

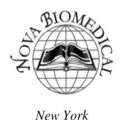

New York

Copyright © 2014 by Nova Science Publishers, Inc.

For permission to use material from this book please contact us:
Telephone 631-231-7269; Fax 631-231-8175
Web Site: http://www.novapublishers.com

NOTICE TO THE READER

The Publisher has taken reasonable care in the preparation of this book, but makes no expressed or implied warranty of any kind and assumes no responsibility for any errors or omissions. No liability is assumed for incidental or consequential damages in connection with or arising out of information contained in this book. The Publisher shall not be liable for any special, consequential, or exemplary damages resulting, in whole or in part, from the readers' use of, or reliance upon, this material. Any parts of this book based on government reports are so indicated and copyright is claimed for those parts to the extent applicable to compilations of such works.

Independent verification should be sought for any data, advice or recommendations contained in this book. In addition, no responsibility is assumed by the publisher for any injury and/or damage to persons or property arising from any methods, products, instructions, ideas or otherwise contained in this publication.

This publication is designed to provide accurate and authoritative information with regard to the subject matter covered herein. It is sold with the clear understanding that the Publisher is not engaged in rendering legal or any other professional services. If legal or any other expert assistance is required, the services of a competent person should be sought. FROM A DECLARATION OF PARTICIPANTS JOINTLY ADOPTED BY A COMMITTEE OF THE AMERICAN BAR ASSOCIATION AND A COMMITTEE OF PUBLISHERS.

Additional color graphics may be available in the e-book version of this book.

Library of Congress Cataloging-in-Publication Data

ISBN: 978-1-63321-037-0

Published by Nova Science Publishers, Inc. † New York

CONTENTS

PREFACE

Chemotherapy is a type of cancer treatment that uses drugs to destroy cancer cells. Chemotherapy works by stopping or slowing the growth of cancer cells, which grow and divide quickly. But it can also harm healthy cells that divide quickly, such as those that line your mouth and intestines or cause your hair to grow. Damage to healthy cells may cause side effects. Often, side effects get better or go away after chemotherapy is over. This book focuses on how patients undergoing chemotherapy can manage their side effects, which symptoms to watch out for, and how to communicate effectively with their health care team. Radiation therapy (also called radiotherapy) is a cancer treatment that uses high doses of radiation to kill cancer cells and stop them from spreading. At low doses, radiation is used as an x-ray to see inside your body and take pictures, such as x-rays of your teeth or broken bones. Radiation used in cancer treatment works in much the same way, except that it is given at higher doses. This book provides facts about radiation therapy and side effects and describes how patients can care for themselves during and after treatment.

Chapter 1 - Chemotherapy and You is written for you—someone who is about to receive or is now receiving chemotherapy for cancer. Your family, friends, and others close to you may also want to read this chapter.

This chapter is a guide you can refer to throughout your chemotherapy treatment. It includes facts about chemotherapy and its side effects and also highlights ways you can care for yourself before, during, and after treatment.

This chapter covers:

- Questions and answers about chemotherapy. Answers common questions, such as what chemotherapy is and how it affects cancer cells.

- Side effects and ways to manage them.
- Explains side effects and other problems that may result from chemotherapy. This section also has ways that you and your doctor or nurse can manage these side effects.
- Tips for meeting with your doctor or nurse.
- Includes questions for you to think about and discuss with your doctor, nurse, and others involved in your cancer care.
- Ways to learn more.
- Lists ways to get more information about chemotherapy and other topics discussed in this chapter—in print, online, and by telephone.
- Words to know.
- A dictionary that clearly explains all the words that are in bold in this chapter.

Talk with your doctor or nurse about what you can expect during chemotherapy.

Chapter 2 - Radiation Therapy and You is written for you—someone who is about to get or is now getting radiation therapy for cancer. People who are close to you may also find this chapter helpful.

This chapter is a guide that you can refer to throughout radiation therapy. It has facts about radiation therapy and side effects and describes how you can care for yourself during and after treatment.

This chapter covers:

- Questions and Answers About Radiation Therapy. Answers to common questions, such as what radiation therapy is and how it affects cancer cells.
- External Beam and Internal Radiation. Information about the two types of radiation therapy.
- Your Feelings During Radiation Therapy. Information about feelings, such as depression and anxiety, and ways to cope with them.
- Side Effects and Ways To Manage Them. A chart that shows problems that may happen as a result of treatment and ways you can help manage them.
- Questions To Ask. Questions for you to think about and discuss with your doctor, nurse, and others involved in your treatment and care.
- Lists of Foods and Liquids. Foods and drinks you can have during radiation therapy.

- Words To Know. A dictionary that clearly explains medical terms used in this chapter. These terms are in bold print the first time they appear.
- Ways To Learn More. Places to go for more information—in print, online (Internet), and by telephone.

Talk with your doctor and nurse about the information in this chapter. They may suggest that you read certain sections or follow some of the tips. Since radiation therapy affects people in different ways, they may also tell you that some of the information in this chapter is not right for you.

In: Cancer Treatment
Editor: Anne E. Wilt

ISBN: 978-1-63321-037-0
© 2014 Nova Science Publishers, Inc.

Chapter 1

CHEMOTHERAPY AND YOU: SUPPORT FOR PEOPLE WITH CANCER[*]

National Cancer Institute

ABOUT THIS CHAPTER

Chemotherapy and You is written for you—someone who is about to receive or is now receiving **chemotherapy** for cancer. Your family, friends, and others close to you may also want to read this chapter.

This chapter is a guide you can refer to throughout your chemotherapy treatment. It includes facts about chemotherapy and its **side effects** and also highlights ways you can care for yourself before, during, and after treatment.

This chapter covers:

- **Questions and answers about chemotherapy.** Answers common questions, such as what chemotherapy is and how it affects cancer cells.
- **Side effects and ways to manage them.**

---

[*] This is an edited, reformatted and augmented version of National Institutes of Health Publication No. 11-7156, revised May 2007.

- Explains side effects and other problems that may result from chemotherapy. This section also has ways that you and your doctor or nurse can manage these side effects.
- **Tips for meeting with your doctor or nurse.**
- Includes questions for you to think about and discuss with your doctor, nurse, and others involved in your cancer care.
- **Ways to learn more.**
- Lists ways to get more information about chemotherapy and other topics discussed in this chapter—in print, online, and by telephone.
- **Words to know.**
- A dictionary that clearly explains all the words that are in bold in this chapter.

Talk with your doctor or nurse about what you can expect during chemotherapy.

QUESTIONS AND ANSWERS ABOUT CHEMOTHERAPY

What Is Chemotherapy?

Chemotherapy (also called chemo) is a type of cancer treatment that uses drugs to destroy cancer cells.

How Does Chemotherapy Work?

Chemotherapy works by stopping or slowing the growth of cancer cells, which grow and divide quickly. But it can also harm **healthy cells** that divide quickly, such as those that line your mouth and intestines or cause your hair to grow. Damage to healthy cells may cause side effects. Often, side effects get better or go away after chemotherapy is over.

What Does Chemotherapy Do?

Depending on your type of cancer and how advanced it is, chemotherapy can:

- **Cure cancer**—when chemotherapy destroys cancer cells to the point that your doctor can no longer detect them in your body and they will not grow back.
- **Control cancer**—when chemotherapy keeps cancer from spreading, slows its growth, or destroys cancer cells that have spread to other parts of your body.
- **Ease cancer symptoms** (also called **palliative care**)—when chemotherapy shrinks tumors that are causing pain or pressure.

How Is Chemotherapy Used?

Sometimes, chemotherapy is used as the only cancer treatment. But more often, you will get chemotherapy along with surgery, **radiation therapy**, or **biological therapy**. Chemotherapy can:

- Make a tumor smaller before surgery or radiation therapy. This is called **neo-adjuvant chemotherapy**.
- Destroy cancer cells that may remain after surgery or radiation therapy. This is called **adjuvant chemotherapy**.
- Help radiation therapy and biological therapy work better.
- Destroy cancer cells that have come back (**recurrent** cancer) or spread to other parts of your body (**metastatic** cancer).

How Does My Doctor Decide Which Chemotherapy Drugs to Use?

This choice depends on:

- The type of cancer you have. Some types of chemotherapy drugs are used for many types of cancer. Other drugs are used for just one or two types of cancer.
- Whether you have had chemotherapy before.
- Whether you have other health problems, such as diabetes or heart disease.

Where Do I Go for Chemotherapy?

You may receive chemotherapy during a hospital stay, at home, or in a doctor's office, clinic, or outpatient unit in a hospital (which means you do not have to stay overnight). No matter where you go for chemotherapy, your doctor and nurse will watch for side effects and make any needed drug changes.

How Often Will I Receive Chemotherapy?

Treatment schedules for chemotherapy vary widely. How often and how long you get chemotherapy depends on:

- Your type of cancer and how advanced it is
- The goals of treatment (whether chemotherapy is used to cure your cancer, control its growth, or ease the symptoms)
- The type of chemotherapy
- How your body reacts to chemotherapy

You may receive chemotherapy in cycles. A cycle is a period of chemotherapy treatment followed by a period of rest. For instance, you might receive 1 week of chemotherapy followed by 3 weeks of rest. These 4 weeks make up one cycle. The rest period gives your body a chance to build new healthy cells.

Can I Miss a Dose of Chemotherapy?

It is not good to skip a chemotherapy treatment. But sometimes your doctor or nurse may change your chemotherapy schedule. This can be due to side effects you are having. If this happens, your doctor or nurse will explain what to do and when to start treatment again.

How Is Chemotherapy Given?

Chemotherapy may be given in many ways.

- **Injection**. The chemotherapy is given by a shot in a muscle in your arm, thigh, or hip, or right under the skin in the fatty part of your arm, leg, or belly.
- **Intra-arterial (IA)**. The chemotherapy goes directly into the artery that is feeding the cancer.
- **Intraperitoneal (IP)**. The chemotherapy goes directly into the **peritoneal cavity** (the area that contains organs such as your intestines, stomach, liver, and ovaries).
- **Intravenous (IV)**. The chemotherapy goes directly into a vein.
- **Topical.** The chemotherapy comes in a cream that you rub onto your skin.
- **Oral**. The chemotherapy comes in pills, capsules, or liquids that you swallow.

Things to Know About Getting Chemotherapy through an IV

Chemotherapy is often given through a thin needle that is placed in a vein on your hand or lower arm. Your nurse will put the needle in at the start of each treatment and remove it when treatment is over. Let your doctor or nurse know right away if you feel pain or burning while you are getting IV chemotherapy.

IV chemotherapy is often given through **catheters** or **ports**, sometimes with the help of a **pump**.

- **Catheters.** A catheter is a soft, thin tube. A surgeon places one end of the catheter in a large vein, often in your chest area. The other end of the catheter stays outside your body. Most catheters stay in place until all your chemotherapy treatments are done. Catheters can also be used for drugs other than chemotherapy and to draw blood. Be sure to watch for signs of infection around your catheter.
- **Ports.** A port is a small, round disc made of plastic or metal that is placed under your skin. A catheter connects the port to a large vein, most often in your chest. Your nurse can insert a needle into your port to give you chemotherapy or draw blood. This needle can be left in place for chemotherapy treatments that are given for more than 1 day. Be sure to watch for signs of infection around your port.
- **Pumps.** Pumps are often attached to catheters or ports. They control how much and how fast chemotherapy goes into a catheter or port.

Pumps can be internal or external. External pumps remain outside your body. Most people can carry these pumps with them. Internal pumps are placed under your skin during surgery.

How Will I Feel During Chemotherapy?

Chemotherapy affects people in different ways. How you feel depends on how healthy you are before treatment, your type of cancer, how advanced it is, the kind of chemotherapy you are getting, and the dose. Doctors and nurses cannot know for certain how you will feel during chemotherapy.

Some people do not feel well right after chemotherapy. The most common side effect is **fatigue**, feeling exhausted and worn out. You can prepare for fatigue by:

- Asking someone to drive you to and from chemotherapy
- Planning time to rest on the day of and day after chemotherapy
- Getting help with meals and childcare the day of and at least 1 day after chemotherapy

Can I Work during Chemotherapy?

Many people can work during chemotherapy, as long as they match their schedule to how they feel. Whether or not you can work may depend on what kind of work you do. If your job allows, you may want to see if you can work part-time or work from home on days you do not feel well.

Many employers are required by law to change your work schedule to meet your needs during cancer treatment. Talk with your employer about ways to adjust your work during chemotherapy. You can learn more about these laws by talking with a social worker.

Can I Take over-the-Counter and Prescription Drugs While I Get Chemotherapy?

This depends on the type of chemotherapy you get and the other types of drugs you plan to take. Take only drugs that are approved by your doctor or nurse. Tell your doctor or nurse about all the over-the-counter and prescription drugs you take, including laxatives, allergy medicines, cold medicines, pain relievers, aspirin, and ibuprofen.

One way to let your doctor or nurse know about these drugs is by bringing in all your pill bottles. Your doctor or nurse needs to know:

- The name of each drug
- The reason you take it
- How much you take
- How often you take it

Talk to your doctor or nurse before you take any over-the-counter or prescription drugs, vitamins, minerals, dietary supplements, or herbs.

Can I Take Vitamins, Minerals, Dietary Supplements, or Herbs While I Get Chemotherapy?

Some of these products can change how chemotherapy works. For this reason, it is important to tell your doctor or nurse about all the vitamins, minerals, dietary supplements, and herbs that you take before you start chemotherapy. During chemotherapy, talk with your doctor before you take any of these products.

How Will I Know If My Chemotherapy Is Working?

Your doctor will give you physical exams and medical tests (such as blood tests and x-rays). He or she will also ask you how you feel.

You cannot tell if chemotherapy is working based on its side effects. Some people think that severe side effects mean that chemotherapy is working well, or that no side effects mean that chemotherapy is not working. The truth is that side effects have nothing to do with how well chemotherapy is fighting your cancer.

How Much Does Chemotherapy Cost?

It is hard to say how much chemotherapy will cost. It depends on:

- The types and doses of chemotherapy used
- How long and how often chemotherapy is given
- Whether you get chemotherapy at home, in a clinic or office, or during a hospital stay
- The part of the country where you live

Does My Health Insurance Pay for Chemotherapy?

Talk with your health insurance company about what costs it will pay for. Questions to ask include:

- What will my insurance pay for?
- Do I need to call my insurance company before each treatment for it to be covered? Or, does my doctor's office need to call?
- What do I have to pay for?
- Can I see any doctor I want or do I need to choose from a list of preferred providers?
- Do I need a written referral to see a specialist?
- Is there a co-pay (money I have to pay) each time I have an appointment?
- Is there a deductible (certain amount I need to pay) before my insurance pays?
- Where should I get my prescription drugs?
- Does my insurance pay for all my tests and treatments, whether I am an inpatient or outpatient?

How Can I Best Work with My Insurance Plan?

- Read your insurance policy before treatment starts to find out what your plan will and will not pay for.
- Keep records of all your treatment costs and insurance claims.
- Send your insurance company all the paperwork it asks for. This may include receipts from doctors' visits, prescriptions, and lab work. Be sure to also keep copies for your own records.
- As needed, ask for help with the insurance paperwork. You can ask a friend, family member, social worker, or local group such as a senior center.

- If your insurance does not pay for something you think it should, find out why the plan refused to pay. Then talk with your doctor or nurse about what to do next. He or she may suggest ways to appeal the decision or other actions to take.

What Are Clinical Trials and Are They an Option for Me?

Cancer clinical trials (also called cancer treatment studies or research studies) test new treatments for people with cancer. These can be studies of new types of chemotherapy, other types of treatment, or new ways to combine treatments. The goal of all these clinical trials is to find better ways to help people with cancer.

Your doctor or nurse may suggest you take part in a clinical trial. You can also suggest the idea. Before you agree to be in a clinical trial, learn about:

- **Benefits.** All clinical trials offer quality cancer care. Ask how this clinical trial could help you or others. For instance, you may be one of the first people to get a new treatment or drug.
- **Risks.** New treatments are not always better or even as good as **standard treatments**. And even if this new treatment is good, it may not work well for you.
- **Payment.** Your insurance company may or may not pay for treatment that is part of a clinical trial. Before you agree to be in a trial, check with your insurance company to make sure it will pay for this treatment.

Contact the NCI's Cancer Information Service if you are interested in learning more about clinical trials.

TIPS FOR MEETING WITH YOUR DOCTOR OR NURSE

- **Make a list of your questions before each appointment.** Some people keep a "running list" and write down new questions as they think of them. Make sure to have space on this list to write down the answers from your doctor or nurse.

- **Bring a family member or trusted friend to your medical visits.** This person can help you understand what the doctor or nurse says and talk with you about it after the visit is over.
- **Ask all your questions.** There is no such thing as a stupid question. If you do not understand an answer, keep asking until you do.
- **Take notes.** You can write them down or use a tape recorder. Later, you can review your notes and remember what was said.
- **Ask for printed information about your type of cancer and chemotherapy.**
- **Let your doctor or nurse know how much information you want to know, when you want to learn it, and when you have learned enough.** Some people want to learn everything they can about cancer and its treatment. Others only want a little information. The choice is yours.
- **Find out how to contact your doctor or nurse in an emergency.** This includes who to call and where to go.

Questions to Ask

About My Cancer
- What kind of cancer do I have?
- What is the stage of my cancer?

About Chemotherapy
- Why do I need chemotherapy?
- What is the goal of this chemotherapy?
- What are the benefits of chemotherapy?
- What are the risks of chemotherapy?
- Are there other ways to treat my type of cancer?
- What is the standard care for my type of cancer?
- Are there any clinical trials for my type of cancer?

About My Treatment
- How many cycles of chemotherapy will I get? How long is each treatment? How long between treatments?
- What types of chemotherapy will I get?
- How will these drugs be given?
- Where do I go for this treatment?

- How long does each treatment last?
- Should someone drive me to and from treatments?

About Side Effects
- What side effects can I expect right away?
- What side effects can I expect later?
- How serious are these side effects?
- How long will these side effects last?
- Will all the side effects go away when treatment is over?
- What can I do to manage or ease these side effects?
- What can my doctor or nurse do to manage or ease side effects?
- When should I call my doctor or nurse about these side effects?

YOUR FEELINGS DURING CHEMOTHERAPY

At some point during chemotherapy, you may feel:

- Anxious
- Depressed
- Afraid
- Angry
- Frustrated
- Helpless
- Lonely

It is normal to have a wide range of feelings while going through chemotherapy. After all, living with cancer and getting treatment can be stressful. You may also feel fatigue, which can make it harder to cope with your feelings.

How Can I Cope with My Feelings during Chemotherapy?
- **Relax.** Find some quiet time and think of yourself in a favorite place. Breathe slowly or listen to soothing music. This may help you feel calmer and less stressed.
- **Exercise.** Many people find that light exercise helps them feel better. There are many ways for you to exercise, such as walking, riding a bike, and doing yoga. Talk with your doctor or nurse about ways you can exercise.

- **Talk with others.** Talk about your feelings with someone you trust. Choose someone who can focus on you, such as a close friend, family member, chaplain, nurse, or social worker. You may also find it helpful to talk with someone else who is getting chemotherapy.

- **Join a support group.** Cancer support groups provide support for people with cancer. These groups allow you to meet others with the same problems. You will have a chance to talk about your feelings and listen to other people talk about theirs. You can find out how others cope with cancer, chemotherapy, and side effects. Your doctor, nurse, or social worker may know about support groups near where you live. Some support groups also meet online (over the Internet), which can be helpful if you cannot travel.

  Talk to your doctor or nurse about things that worry or upset you. You may want to ask about seeing a counselor. Your doctor may also suggest that you take medication if you find it very hard to cope with your feelings.

It's normal to have a wide range of feelings during chemotherapy. After all, living with cancer and going through treatment can be stressful.

Ways to Learn More

To learn more about coping with your feelings and relationships during cancer treatment, read *Taking Time: Support for People With Cancer*, a book from the National Cancer Institute. You can get a free copy at http://www.cancer.gov/ publications or 1-800-4-CANCER (1-800-422-6237).

Cancer Support Community
Dedicated to providing support, education, and hope to people affected by cancer.
Call: 1-888-793-9355 or 202-659-9709
Visit: http://www.cancersupportcommunity.org
E-mail: help@cancersupportcommunity.org

Cancer*Care*, Inc.
Offers free support, information, financial assistance, and practical help to people with cancer and their loved ones.
Call: 1-800-813-HOPE (1-800-813-4673)

Visit: http://www.cancercare.org
E-mail: info@cancercare.org

SIDE EFFECTS AND WAYS TO MANAGE THEM

What Are Side Effects?

Side effects are problems caused by cancer treatment. Some common side effects from chemotherapy are fatigue, **nausea**, **vomiting**, decreased **blood cell counts**, hair loss, mouth sores, and pain.

What Causes Side Effects?

Chemotherapy is designed to kill fast-growing cancer cells. But it can also affect healthy cells that grow quickly. These include cells that line your mouth and intestines, cells in your bone marrow that make blood cells, and cells that make your hair grow. Chemotherapy causes side effects when it harms these healthy cells.

Will I Get Side Effects from Chemotherapy?

You may have a lot of side effects, some, or none at all. This depends on the type and amount of chemotherapy you get and how your body reacts. Before you start chemotherapy, talk with your doctor or nurse about which side effects to expect.

How Long Do Side Effects Last?

How long side effects last depends on your health and the kind of chemotherapy you get. Most side effects go away after chemotherapy is over. But sometimes it can take months or even years for them to go away.

Sometimes, chemotherapy causes long-term side effects that do not go away. These may include damage to your heart, lungs, nerves, kidneys, or reproductive organs. Some types of chemotherapy may cause a second cancer years later. Ask your doctor or nurse about your chance of having long-term side effects.

What Can Be Done About Side Effects?

Doctors have many ways to prevent or treat chemotherapy side effects and help you heal after each treatment session. Talk with your doctor or nurse about which ones to expect and what to do about them. Make sure to let your doctor or nurse know about any changes you notice—they may be signs of a side effect.

Side Effects at-a-Glance

Below is a list of side effects that chemotherapy may cause.

Not everyone gets every side effect. Which ones you have will depend on the type and dose of your chemotherapy and whether you have other health problems, such as diabetes or heart disease.

Talk with your doctor or nurse about the side effects on this list.

Side effects
Anemia
Appetite changes
Bleeding
Constipation
Diarrhea
Fatigue
Flu-like symptoms
Fluid retention
Hair loss
Infection
Infertility
Mouth and throat changes
Nausea and vomiting
Nervous system changes
Pain
Sexual changes

| Skin and nail changes |
| Eye changes |
| Urinary, kidney, and bladder changes |

Anemia

What It Is and Why It Occurs

Red blood cells carry oxygen throughout your body. **Anemia** is when you have too few red blood cells to carry the oxygen your body needs. Your heart works harder when your body does not get enough oxygen. This can make it feel like your heart is pounding or beating very fast. Anemia can also make you feel short of breath, weak, dizzy, faint, or very tired.

Some types of chemotherapy cause anemia because they make it harder for bone marrow to produce new red blood cells.

Ways to Manage

- **Get plenty of rest.** Try to sleep at least 8 hours each night. You might also want to take 1 to 2 short naps (1 hour or less) during the day.
- **Limit your activities.** This means doing only the activities that are most important to you. For example, you might go to work but not clean the house. Or you might order takeout food instead of cooking dinner.
- **Accept help.** When your family or friends offer to help, let them. They can help care for your children, pick up groceries, run errands, drive you to doctor's visits, or do other chores you feel too tired to do.
- **Eat a well-balanced diet.** Choose a diet that contains all the calories and protein your body needs. Calories will help keep your weight up, and extra protein can help repair tissues that have been harmed by cancer treatment. Talk to your doctor, nurse, or dietitian about the diet that is right for you.
- **Stand up slowly.** You may feel dizzy if you stand up too fast. When you get up from lying down, sit for a minute before you stand.

Your doctor or nurse will check your blood cell count throughout your chemotherapy. You may need a blood transfusion if your red blood cell count falls too low. Your doctor may also prescribe a medicine to boost (speed up) the growth of red blood cells or suggest that you take iron or other vitamins.

Call your doctor or nurse if:

- Your level of fatigue changes or you are not able to do your usual activities
- You feel dizzy or like you are going to faint
- You feel short of breath
- It feels like your heart is pounding or beating very fast

Appetite Changes

What They Are and Why They Occur
Chemotherapy can cause appetite changes. You may lose your appetite because of nausea (feeling like you are going to throw up), mouth and throat problems that make it painful to eat, or drugs that cause you to lose your taste for food. The changes can also come from feeling depressed or tired. Appetite loss may last for a day, a few weeks, or even months.

It is important to eat well, even when you have no appetite. This means eating and drinking foods that have plenty of protein, vitamins, and calories. Eating well helps your body fight infection and repair tissues that are damaged by chemotherapy. Not eating well can lead to weight loss, weakness, and fatigue.

Some cancer treatments cause weight gain or an increase in your appetite. Be sure to ask your doctor, nurse, or dietitian what types of appetite changes you might expect and how to manage them.

Ways to Manage
- **Eat 5 to 6 small meals or snacks each day instead of 3 big meals.** Choose foods and drinks that are high in calories and protein.
- **Set a daily schedule for eating your meals and snacks.** Eat when it is time to eat, rather than when you feel hungry. You may not feel hungry while you are on chemotherapy, but you still need to eat.
- **Drink milkshakes, smoothies, juice, or soup if you do not feel like eating solid foods.** Liquids like these can help provide the protein, vitamins, and calories your body needs.
- **Use plastic forks and spoons.** Some types of chemo give you a metal taste in your mouth. Eating with plastic can help decrease the metal taste. Cooking in glass pots and pans can also help.

- **Increase your appetite by doing something active.** For instance, you might have more of an appetite if you take a short walk before lunch. Also, be careful not to decrease your appetite by drinking too much liquid before or during meals.
- **Change your routine.** This may mean eating in a different place, such as the dining room rather than the kitchen. It can also mean eating with other people instead of eating alone. If you eat alone, you may want to listen to the radio or watch TV. You may also want to vary your diet by trying new foods and recipes.
- **Talk with your doctor, nurse, or dietitian**. He or she may want you to take extra vitamins or nutrition supplements (such as high protein drinks). If you cannot eat for a long time and are losing weight, you may need to take drugs that increase your appetite or receive nutrition through an IV or feeding tube.

NCI's book "Eating Hints: BeFore, During, and After Cancer Treatment" provides more tips For making eating easier.

You can get a Free copy at http://www.cancer or 1-B00-4-CANCER (1-B00-422-6237).

Bleeding

What It Is and Why It Occurs

Platelets are cells that make your blood clot when you bleed. Chemotherapy can lower the number of platelets because it affects your bone marrow's ability to make them. A low platelet count is called **thrombocytopenia**. This condition may cause bruises (even when you have not been hit or have not bumped into anything), bleeding from your nose or in your mouth, or a rash of tiny, red dots.

Ways to Manage

Do:

- Brush your teeth with a very soft toothbrush
- Soften the bristles of your toothbrush by running hot water over them before you brush
- Blow your nose gently
- Be careful when using scissors, knives, or other sharp objects

- Use an electric shaver instead of a razor
- Apply gentle but firm pressure to any cuts you get until the bleeding stops
- Wear shoes all the time, even inside the house or hospital

Do not:
- Use dental floss or toothpicks
- Play sports or do other activities during which you could get hurt
- Use tampons, enemas, suppositories, or rectal thermometers
- Wear clothes with tight collars, wrists, or waistbands

Check with Your Doctor or Nurse Before:
- Drinking beer, wine, or other types of alcohol
- Having sex
- Taking vitamins, herbs, minerals, dietary supplements, aspirin, or other over-the-counter medicines. Some of these products can change how chemotherapy works.

Check with your doctor or nurse before taking any vitamins, herbs, minerals, dietary supplements, aspirin, or other over-the-counter medicines.

Let Your Doctor Know if You Are Constipated
He or she may prescribe a stool softener to prevent straining and rectal bleeding when you go to the bathroom.

Your Doctor or Nurse Will Check Your Platelet Count Often
You may need medication, a platelet transfusion, or a delay in your chemotherapy treatment if your platelet count is too low.

Call Your Doctor or Nurse if You Have Any of These Symptoms
- Bruises, especially if you did not bump into anything
- Small, red spots on your skin
- Red- or pink-colored urine
- Black or bloody bowel movements
- Bleeding from your gums or nose
- Heavy bleeding during your menstrual period or for a prolonged period
- Vaginal bleeding not caused by your period

- Headaches or changes in your vision
- A warm or hot feeling in your arm or leg
- Feeling very sleepy or confused

Constipation

What It Is and Why It Occurs

Constipation is when bowel movements become less frequent and stools are hard, dry, and difficult to pass. You may have painful bowel movements and feel bloated or nauseous. You may belch, pass a lot of gas, and have stomach cramps or pressure in the rectum.

Drugs such as chemotherapy and pain medicine can cause constipation. It can also happen when people are not active and spend a lot of time sitting or lying down. Constipation can also be due to eating foods that are low in fiber or not drinking enough fluids.

Ways to Manage

- **Keep a record of your bowel movements.** Show this record to your doctor or nurse and talk about what is normal for you. This makes it easier to figure out whether you have constipation.
- **Drink at least 8 cups of water or other fluids each day.** Many people find that drinking warm or hot fluids, such as coffee and tea, helps with constipation. Fruit juices, such as prune juice, may also be helpful.

When you eat more fiber, be sure to drink more fluids.

- **Be active every day.** You can be active by walking, riding a bike, or doing yoga. If you cannot walk, ask about exercises that you can do in a chair or bed. Talk with your doctor or nurse about ways you can be more active.

Check with your doctor or nurse before using fiber supplements, laxatives, stool softeners, or enemas.

- **Ask your doctor, nurse, or dietitian about foods that are high in fiber.** Eating high-fiber foods and drinking lots of fluids can help soften your stools. Good sources of fiber include whole-grain breads

and cereals, dried beans and peas, raw vegetables, fresh and dried
fruit, nuts, seeds, and popcorn.
• **Let your doctor or nurse know if you have not had a bowel
  movement in 2 days.** Your doctor may suggest a fiber supplement,
  laxative, stool softener, or enema. Do not use these treatments without
  first checking with your doctor or nurse.

Diarrhea

What It Is and Why It Occurs
Diarrhea is frequent bowel movements that may be soft, loose, or watery.
Chemotherapy can cause diarrhea because it harms healthy cells that line your
large and small intestines. It may also speed up your bowels. Diarrhea can also
be caused by infections or drugs used to treat constipation.

Ways to Manage
• **Eat 5 or 6 small meals and snacks each day instead of 3 large
  meals.**
• **Ask your doctor or nurse about foods that are high in salts such
  as sodium and potassium.** Your body can lose these salts when you
  have diarrhea, and it is important to replace them. Foods that are high
  in sodium or potassium include bananas, oranges, peach and apricot
  nectar, and boiled or mashed potatoes.
• **Drink 8 to 12 cups of clear liquids each day.** These include water,
  clear broth, ginger ale, or sports drinks such as Gatorade® or
  Propel®. Drink slowly, and choose drinks that are at room
  temperature. Let carbonated drinks lose their fizz before you drink
  them. Add extra water if drinks make you thirsty or nauseous (feeling
  like you are going to throw up).
• **Eat low-fiber foods.** Foods that are high in fiber can make diarrhea
  worse. Low-fiber foods include bananas, white rice, white toast, and
  plain or vanilla yogurt.
• **Let your doctor or nurse know if your diarrhea lasts for more
  than 24 hours or if you have pain and cramping along with
  diarrhea. Your doctor may prescribe a medicine to control the
  diarrhea.** You may also need IV fluids to replace the water and
  nutrients you lost. Do not take any medicine for diarrhea without first
  asking your doctor or nurse.

Ask your doctor or nurse beFore taking medicine For diarrhea.

- **Be gentle when you wipe yourself after a bowel movement.** Instead of toilet paper, use a baby wipe or squirt of water from a spray bottle to clean yourself after bowel movements. Let your doctor or nurse know if your rectal area is sore or bleeds or if you have hemorrhoids.
- **Ask your doctor if you should try a clear liquid diet.** This can give your bowels time to rest. Most people stay on this type of diet for 5 days or less.

Stay away from:

- Drinks that are very hot or very cold
- Beer, wine, and other types of alcohol
- Milk or milk products, such as ice cream, milkshakes, sour cream, and cheese
- Spicy foods, such as hot sauce, salsa, chili, and curry dishes
- Greasy and fried foods, such as french fries and hamburgers
- Foods or drinks with caffeine, such as regular coffee, black tea, cola, and chocolate
- Foods or drinks that cause gas, such as cooked dried beans, cabbage, broccoli, and soy milk and other soy products
- Foods that are high in fiber, such as cooked dried beans, raw fruits and vegetables, nuts, and whole-wheat breads and cereals

To learn more about ways to manage diarrhea during cancer treatment read *Eating Hints: Before, During, and After Cancer Treatment*, a book from NCI. You can get a free copy at http://www.cancer.gov/publications or by calling 1-800-4-CANCER (1-800-422-6237).

Fatigue

What It Is and Why It Occurs

Fatigue from chemotherapy can range from a mild to extreme feeling of being tired. Many people describe fatigue as feeling weak, weary, worn out, heavy, or slow. Resting does not always help.

Many people say they feel fatigue during chemotherapy and even for weeks or months after treatment is over. Fatigue can be caused by the type of chemotherapy, the effort of making frequent visits to the doctor, or feelings such as stress, anxiety, and depression. If you receive radiation therapy along with chemotherapy, your fatigue may be more severe.

Fatigue can also be caused by:

- Anemia
- Pain
- Medications
- Appetite changes
- Trouble sleeping
- Lack of activity
- Trouble breathing
- Infection
- Doing too much at one time
- Other medical problems

Fatigue can happen all at once or little by little. People feel fatigue in different ways. You may feel more or less fatigue than someone else who gets the same type of chemotherapy.

Ways to manage
- **Relax.** You might want to try meditation, prayer, yoga, guided imagery, visualization, or other ways to relax and decrease stress.
- **Eat and drink well.** Often, this means 5 to 6 small meals and snacks rather than 3 large meals. Keep foods around that are easy to fix, such as canned soups, frozen meals, yogurt, and cottage cheese. Drink plenty of fluids each day—about 8 cups of water or juice.
- **Plan time to rest.** You may feel better when you rest or take a short nap during the day. Many people say that it helps to rest for just 10 to 15 minutes rather than nap for a long time. If you nap, try to sleep for less than 1 hour. Keeping naps short will help you sleep better at night.
- **Be active.** Research shows that exercise can ease fatigue and help you sleep better at night. Try going for a 15-minute walk, doing yoga, or riding an exercise bike. Plan to be active when you have the most energy. Talk with your doctor or nurse about ways you can be active while getting chemotherapy.
- **Try not to do too much.** With fatigue, you may not have enough energy to do all the things you want to do. Choose the activities you

want to do and let someone else help with the others. Try quiet activities, such as reading, knitting, or learning a new language on tape.

- **Sleep at least 8 hours each night.** This may be more sleep than you needed before chemotherapy. You are likely to sleep better at night when you are active during the day. You may also find it helpful to relax before going to bed. For instance, you might read a book, work on a jigsaw puzzle, listen to music, or do other quiet hobbies.

- **Plan a work schedule that works for you.** Fatigue may affect the amount of energy you have for your job. You may feel well enough to work your full schedule. Or you may need to work less—maybe just a few hours a day or a few days each week. If your job allows, you may want to talk with your boss about ways to work from home. Or you may want to go on medical leave (stop working for a while) while getting chemotherapy.

- **Let others help.** Ask family members and friends to help when you feel fatigue. Perhaps they can help with household chores or drive you to and from doctor's visits. They might also help by shopping for food and cooking meals for you to eat now or freeze for later.

- **Learn from others who have cancer.** People who have cancer can help by sharing ways that they manage fatigue. One way to meet others is by joining a support group—either in person or online. Talk with your doctor or nurse to learn more.

- **Keep a diary of how you feel each day.** This will help you plan how to best use your time. Share your diary with your nurse. Let your doctor or nurse know if you notice changes in your energy level, whether you have lots of energy or are very tired.

- **Talk with your doctor or nurse.** Your doctor may prescribe medication that can help decrease fatigue, give you a sense of well-being, and increase your appetite. He or she may also suggest treatment if your fatigue is from anemia.

Hair Loss

What It Is and Why It Occurs

Hair loss (also called **alopecia**) is when some or all of your hair falls out. This can happen anywhere on your body: your head, face, arms, legs, underarms, or the pubic area between your legs. Many people are upset by the loss of their hair and find it the most difficult part of chemotherapy.

Some types of chemotherapy damage the cells that cause hair growth. Hair loss often starts 2 to 3 weeks after chemotherapy begins. Your scalp may hurt at first. Then you may lose your hair, either a little at a time or in clumps. It takes about 1 week for all your hair to fall out. Almost always, your hair will grow back 2 to 3 months after chemotherapy is over. You may notice that your hair starts growing back even while you are getting chemotherapy.

Your hair will be very fine when it starts growing back. Also, your new hair may not look or feel the same as it did before. For instance, your hair may be thin instead of thick, curly instead of straight, and darker or lighter in color.

Hair oFten grows back 2 to 3 months aFter chemotherapy is over.

Ways to Manage
Before hair loss:

- **Talk with your doctor or nurse.** He or she will know if you are likely to have hair loss.
- **Cut your hair short or shave your head.** You might feel more in control of hair loss if you first cut your hair or shave your head. This often makes hair loss easier to manage. If you shave your head, use an electric shaver instead of a razor.

IF you plan to buy a wig, do so while you still have hair.

- **The best time to choose your wig is before chemotherapy starts.** This way, you can match the wig to the color and style of your hair. You might also take it to your hair dresser who can style the wig to look like your own hair. Make sure to choose a wig that feels comfortable and does not hurt your scalp.
- **Ask if your insurance company will pay for a wig.** If it will not, you can deduct the cost of your wig as a medical expense on your income tax. Some groups also have free "wig banks." Your doctor, nurse, or social worker will know if there is a wig bank near you.
- **Be gentle when you wash your hair.** Use a mild shampoo, such as a baby shampoo. Dry your hair by patting (not rubbing) it with a soft towel.
- **Do not use items that can hurt your scalp.** These include:

- Straightening or curling irons
- Brush rollers or curlers
- Electric hair dryers
- Hair bands and clips
- Hairsprays
- Hair dyes
- Products to perm or relax your hair

After hair loss:

- **Protect your scalp.** Your scalp may hurt during and after hair loss. Protect it by wearing a hat, turban, or scarf when you are outside. Try to avoid places that are very hot or very cold. This includes tanning beds and outside in the sun or cold air. And always apply sunscreen or sunblock to protect your scalp.
- **Stay warm.** You may feel colder once you lose your hair. Wear a hat, turban, scarf, or wig to help you stay warm.
- **Sleep on a satin pillow case.** Satin creates less friction than cotton when you sleep on it. Therefore, you may find satin pillow cases more comfortable.
- **Talk about your feelings.** Many people feel angry, depressed, or embarrassed about hair loss. If you are very worried or upset, you might want to talk about these feelings with a doctor, nurse, family member, close friend, or someone who has had hair loss caused by cancer treatment.

Ways to learn more
American Cancer Society
Offers a variety of services to people with cancer and their families, including referrals to low-cost wig banks.
Call: 1-800-ACS-2345 (1-800-227-2345)
TTY: 1-866-228-4327; Visit: http://www.cancer

Infection

What It Is and Why It Occurs
Some types of chemotherapy make it harder for your bone marrow to produce new **white blood cells**. White blood cells help your body fight

infection. Therefore, it is important to avoid infections, since chemotherapy decreases the number of your white blood cells.

There are many types of white blood cells. One type is called **neutrophil**. When your neutrophil count is low, it is called **neutropenia**. Your doctor or nurse may do blood tests to find out whether you have neutropenia.

It is important to watch for signs of infection when you have neutropenia. Check for fever at least once a day, or as often as your doctor or nurse tells you to. You may find it best to use a digital thermometer. Call your doctor or nurse if your temperature is 100.5°F or higher.

Call your doctor or nurse right away if you have a fever of 100.5°F or higher.

Ways to manage

- **Your doctor or nurse will check your white blood cell count throughout your treatment.** If chemotherapy is likely to make your white blood cell count very low, you may get medicine to raise your white blood cell count and lower your risk of infection.
- **Wash your hands often with soap and water.** Be sure to wash your hands before cooking and eating, and after you use the bathroom, blow your nose, cough, sneeze, or touch animals. Carry hand sanitizer for times when you are not near soap and water.
- **Use sanitizing wipes to clean surfaces and items that you touch.** This includes public telephones, ATM machines, doorknobs, and other common items.
- **Be gentle and thorough when you wipe yourself after a bowel movement.** Instead of toilet paper, use a baby wipe or squirt of water from a spray bottle to clean yourself. Let your doctor or nurse know if your rectal area is sore or bleeds or if you have hemorrhoids.
- **Stay away from people who are sick.** This includes people with colds, flu, measles, or chicken pox. You also need to stay away from children who just had a "live virus" vaccine for chicken pox or polio. Call your doctor, nurse, or local health department if you have any questions.
- **Stay away from crowds.** Try not to be around a lot of people. For instance, plan to go shopping or to the movies when the stores and theaters are less crowded.

- **Be careful not to cut or nick yourself.** Do not cut or tear your nail cuticles. Use an electric shaver instead of a razor. And be extra careful when using scissors, needles, or knives.
- **Watch for signs of infection around your catheter.** Signs include drainage, redness, swelling, or soreness. Let your doctor or nurse know about any changes you notice near your catheter.
- **Maintain good mouth care.** Brush your teeth after meals and before you go to bed. Use a very soft toothbrush. You can make the bristles even softer by running hot water over them just before you brush. Use a mouth rinse that does not contain alcohol. Check with your doctor or nurse before going to the dentist.
- **Take good care of your skin.** Do not squeeze or scratch pimples. Use lotion to soften and heal dry, cracked skin. Dry yourself after a bath or shower by gently patting (not rubbing) your skin.
- **Clean cuts right away.** Use warm water, soap, and an antiseptic to clean your cuts. Do this every day until your cut has a scab over it.
- **Be careful around animals.** Do not clean your cat's litter box, pick up dog waste, or clean bird cages or fish tanks. Be sure to wash your hands after touching pets and other animals.
- **Do not get a flu shot or other type of vaccine without first asking your doctor or nurse.** Some vaccines contain a live virus, which you should not be exposed to.
- **Keep hot foods hot and cold foods cold.** Do not leave leftovers sitting out. Put them in the refrigerator as soon as you are done eating.
- **Wash raw vegetables and fruits well before eating them.**
- **Do not eat raw or undercooked fish, seafood, meat, chicken, or eggs.** These may have bacteria that can cause infection.
- **Do not have food or drinks that are moldy, spoiled, or past the freshness date.**

Do not take drugs that reduce fever without first talking with your doctor or nurse.

- **Call your doctor right away (even on the weekend or in the middle of the night) if you think you have an infection.** Be sure you know how to reach your doctor after office hours and on weekends. Call if you have a fever of 100.5°F or higher, or when you have chills or sweats. Do not take aspirin, acetaminophen (such as Tylenol®), ibuprofen products, or any other drugs that reduce fever without first talking with your doctor or nurse. Other signs of infection include:

- Redness
- Swelling
- Rash
- Chills
- Cough
- Earache
- Headache
- Stiff neck
- Bloody or cloudy urine
- Painful or frequent need to urinate
- Sinus pain or pressure

Infertility

What It Is and Why It Occurs

Some types of chemotherapy can cause **infertility**. For a woman, this means that you may not be able to get pregnant. For a man, this means you may not be able to get a woman pregnant.

In women, chemotherapy may damage the ovaries. This damage can lower the number of healthy eggs in the ovaries. It can also lower the **hormones** produced by them. The drop in hormones can lead to early menopause. Early menopause and fewer healthy eggs can cause infertility.

In men, chemotherapy may damage sperm cells, which grow and divide quickly. Infertility may occur because chemotherapy can lower the number of sperm, make sperm less able to move, or cause other types of damage.

Whether or not you become infertile depends on the type of chemotherapy you get, your age, and whether you have other health problems. Infertility can last the rest of your life.

Before treatment starts, tell your doctor or nurse iF you want to have children in the Future.

Ways to Manage
For WOMEN, talk with your doctor or nurse about:

- Whether you want to have children. Before you start chemotherapy, let your doctor or nurse know if you might want to get pregnant in the future. He or she may talk with you about ways to preserve your eggs to use after treatment ends or refer you to a fertility specialist.
- Birth control. It is very important that you do not get pregnant while getting chemotherapy. These drugs can hurt the fetus, especially in the first 3 months of pregnancy. If you have not yet gone through menopause, talk with your doctor or nurse about birth control and ways to keep from getting pregnant.
- Pregnancy. If you still have menstrual periods, your doctor or nurse may ask you to have a pregnancy test before you start chemotherapy. If you are pregnant, your doctor or nurse will talk with you about other treatment options.

Chemotherapy can cause birth deFects. Po not get pregnant while you are getting treatment.

Talk with your doctor or nurse about saving your sperm beFore you start treatment, iF you want to Father children in the Future.

For MEN, talk with your doctor or nurse about:

- **Whether you want to have children.** Before you start chemotherapy, let your doctor or nurse know if you might want to father children in the future. He or she may talk with you about ways to preserve your sperm to use in the future or refer you to a fertility specialist.
- **Birth control.** It is very important that your spouse or partner does not get pregnant while you are getting chemotherapy. Chemotherapy can damage your sperm and cause birth defects.

Chemotherapy may damage sperm and cause birth deFects. Make sure that your spouse or partner does not get pregnant while you are in treatment.

Ways to Learn More

American Cancer Society
Offers a variety of services to people with cancer and their families.
Call: 1-800-ACS-2345 (1-800-227-2345)
TTY: 1-866-228-4327
Visit: http://www.cancer

fertileHOPE

A LIVESTRONG initiative dedicated to providing reproductive information, support, and hope to cancer patients and survivors whose medical treatments present the risk of infertility.

Call: 1-866-965-7205

Visit: http://www.fertilehope.org

Mouth and Throat Changes

What They Are and Why They Occur

Some types of chemotherapy harm fast-growing cells, such as those that line your mouth, throat, and lips. This can affect your teeth, gums, the lining of your mouth, and the glands that make saliva. Most mouth problems go away a few days after chemotherapy is over.

Mouth and throat problems may include:
- Dry mouth (having little or no saliva)
- Changes in taste and smell (such as when food tastes like metal or chalk, has no taste, or does not taste or smell like it used to)
- Infections of your gums, teeth, or tongue
- Increased sensitivity to hot or cold foods
- Mouth sores
- Trouble eating when your mouth gets very sore

Ways to Manage
- **Visit a dentist at least 2 weeks before starting chemotherapy.** It is important to have your mouth as healthy as possible. This means getting all your dental work done before chemotherapy starts. If you cannot go to the dentist before chemotherapy starts, ask your doctor or nurse when it is safe to go. Be sure to tell your dentist that you have cancer and about your treatment plan.
- **Check your mouth and tongue every day.** This way, you can see or feel problems (such as mouth sores, white spots, or infections) as soon as they start. Inform your doctor or nurse about these problems right away.

Visit your dentist at least 2 weeks before starting chemotherapy.

- **Keep your mouth moist.** You can keep your mouth moist by sipping water throughout the day, sucking on ice chips or sugar-free hard candy, or chewing sugar-free gum. Ask your doctor or nurse about saliva substitutes if your mouth is always dry.
- **Clean your mouth, teeth, gums, and tongue.**
  - Brush your teeth, gums, and tongue after each meal and at bedtime.
  - Use an extra-soft toothbrush. You can make the bristles even softer by rinsing your toothbrush in hot water before you brush.
  - If brushing is painful, try cleaning your teeth with cotton swabs or Toothettes®.
  - Use a fluoride toothpaste or special fluoride gel that your dentist prescribes.
  - Do not use mouthwash that has alcohol. Instead, rinse your mouth 3 to 4 times a day with a solution of 1/4 teaspoon baking soda and 1/8 teaspoon salt in 1 cup of warm water. Follow this with a plain water rinse.
  - Gently floss your teeth every day. If your gums bleed or hurt, avoid those areas but floss your other teeth. Ask your doctor or nurse about flossing if your platelet count is low.
  - If you wear dentures, make sure they fit well and keep them clean. Also, limit the length of time that you wear them.
- **Be careful what you eat when your mouth is sore.**
  - Choose foods that are moist, soft, and easy to chew or swallow. These include cooked cereals, mashed potatoes, and scrambled eggs.
  - Use a blender to puree cooked foods so that they are easier to eat. To help avoid infection, be sure to wash all blender parts before and after using them. If possible, it is best to wash them in a dishwasher.
  - Take small bites of food, chew slowly, and sip liquids while you eat.
  - Soften food with gravy, sauces, broth, yogurt, or other liquids.
  - Eat foods that are cool or at room temperature. You may find that warm and hot foods hurt your mouth or throat.
  - Suck on ice chips or popsicles. These can relieve mouth pain.
  - Ask your dietitian for ideas of foods that are easy to eat.

Call your doctor, nurse, or dentist if your mouth hurts a lot. Your doctor or dentist may prescribe medicine for pain or to keep your mouth moist. Make sure to give your dentist the phone number of your doctor and nurse.

- **Stay away from things that can hurt, scrape, or burn your mouth, such as:**
  - Sharp or crunchy foods, such as crackers and potato or corn chips
  - Spicy foods, such as hot sauce, curry dishes, salsa, and chili
  - Citrus fruits or juices such as orange, lemon, and grapefruit
  - Food and drinks that have a lot of sugar, such as candy or soda
  - Beer, wine, and other types of alcohol
  - Toothpicks or other sharp objects
  - Tobacco products, including cigarettes, pipes, cigars, and chewing tobacco

Do not use tobacco or drink alcohol if your mouth is sore.

Ways to Learn More
National Oral Health Information Clearinghouse
A service of the National Institutes of Dental and Craniofacial Research that provides oral health information for special care patients.
Call: 1-866-232-4528
Visit: http://www.nidcr.nih.gov
E-mail: nidcrinfo@mail.nih.gov

Smokefree.gov
Provides resources including information on quitlines, a step-by-step cessation guide, and publications to help you or someone you care about quit smoking.
Call: 1-877-44U-QUIT (1-877-448-7848)
Visit: http://www.smokefree.gov

Nausea and Vomiting

What They Are and Why They Occur
Some types of chemotherapy can cause nausea, vomiting, or both. Nausea is when you feel sick to your stomach, like you are going to throw up.

Vomiting is when you throw up. You may also have **dry heaves**, which is when your body tries to vomit even though your stomach is empty.

Nausea and vomiting can occur while you are getting chemotherapy, right after, or many hours or days later. You will most likely feel better on the days you do not get chemotherapy.

New drugs can help prevent nausea and vomiting. These are called **antiemetic** or **antinausea** drugs. You may need to take these drugs 1 hour before each chemotherapy treatment and for a few days after. How long you take them after chemotherapy will depend on the type of chemotherapy you are getting and how you react to it. If one antinausea drug does not work well for you, your doctor can prescribe a different one. You may need to take more than one type of drug to help with nausea. **Acupuncture** may also help. Talk with your doctor or nurse about treatments to control nausea and vomiting caused by chemotherapy.

Ways to Manage
- **Prevent nausea.** One way to prevent vomiting is to prevent nausea. Try having bland, easy-to-digest foods and drinks that do not upset your stomach. These include plain crackers, toast, and gelatin.
- **Plan when it's best for you to eat and drink.** Some people feel better when they eat a light meal or snack before chemotherapy. Others feel better when they have chemotherapy on an empty stomach (nothing to eat or drink for 2 to 3 hours before treatment). After treatment, wait at least 1 hour before you eat or drink.
- **Eat small meals and snacks.** Instead of 3 large meals each day, you might feel better if you eat 5 or 6 small meals and snacks. Do not drink a lot before or during meals. Also, do not lie down right after you eat.
- **Have foods and drinks that are warm or cool (not hot or cold).** Give hot foods and drinks time to cool down, or make them colder by adding ice. You can warm up cold foods by taking them out of the refrigerator 1 hour before you eat or warming them slightly in a microwave. Drink cola or ginger ale that is warm and has lost its fizz.

Eat 5 or 6 small meals and snacks each day instead of 3 large ones.

- **Stay away from foods and drinks with strong smells.** These include coffee, fish, onions, garlic, and foods that are cooking.

- **Try small bites of popsicles or fruit ices.** You may also find sucking on ice chips helpful.
- **Suck on sugar-free mints or tart candies.** But do not use tart candies if you have mouth or throat sores.
- **Relax before treatment.** You may feel less nausea if you relax before each chemotherapy treatment. Meditate, do deep breathing exercises, or imagine scenes or experiences that make you feel peaceful. You can also do quiet hobbies such as reading, listening to music, or knitting.
- **When you feel like vomiting, breathe deeply and slowly or get fresh air.** You might also distract yourself by chatting with friends or family, listening to music, or watching a movie or TV.
- **Talk with your doctor or nurse.** Your doctor can give you drugs to help prevent nausea during and after chemotherapy. Be sure to take these drugs as ordered and let your doctor or nurse know if they do not work. You might also ask your doctor or nurse about acupuncture, which can help relieve nausea and vomiting caused by cancer treatment.

Tell your doctor or nurse if you vomit for more than 1 day or right after you drink.

Let your doctor or nurse know iF your medicine For nausea is not working.

To learn more about dealing with nausea and vomiting during cancer treatment read *Eating Hints: Before, During, and After Cancer Treatment*, a book from NCI. You can get a free copy at http://www.cancer.gov /publications or by calling 1-800-4-CANCER (1-800-422-6237).

Nervous System Changes

What They Are and Why They Occur
Chemotherapy can cause damage to your nervous system. Many nervous system problems get better within a year of when you finish chemotherapy, but some may last the rest of your life. Symptoms may include:

- Tingling, burning, weakness, or numbness in your hands or feet
- Feeling colder than normal

- Pain when walking
- Weak, sore, tired, or achy muscles
- Being clumsy and losing your balance
- Trouble picking up objects or buttoning your clothes
- Shaking or trembling
- Hearing loss
- Stomach pain, such as constipation or heartburn
- Fatigue
- Confusion and memory problems
- Dizziness
- Depression

Let your doctor or nurse know right away if you notice any nervous system changes. It is important to treat these problems as soon as possible.

Ways to Manage

- **Let your doctor or nurse know right away if you notice any nervous system changes.** It is important to treat these problems as soon as possible.
- **Be careful when handling knives, scissors, and other sharp or dangerous objects.**
- **Avoid falling.** Walk slowly, hold onto handrails when using the stairs, and put no-slip bath mats in your bathtub or shower. Make sure there are no area rugs or cords to trip over.
- **Always wear sneakers, tennis shoes, or other footwear with rubber soles.**
- **Check the temperature of your bath water with a thermometer.** This will keep you from getting burned by water that is too hot.
- **Be extra careful to avoid burning or cutting yourself while cooking.**
- **Wear gloves when working in the garden, cooking, or washing dishes.**
- **Rest when you need to.**
- **Steady yourself when you walk by using a cane or other device.**
- **Talk to your doctor or nurse if you notice memory problems, feel confused, or are depressed.**
- **Ask your doctor for pain medicine if you need it.**

Pain

What It Is and Why It Occurs

Some types of chemotherapy cause painful side effects. These include burning, numbness, and tingling or shooting pains in your hands and feet. Mouth sores, headaches, muscle pains, and stomach pains can also occur.

Pain can be caused by the cancer itself or by chemotherapy. Doctors and nurses have ways to decrease or relieve your pain.

Be sure to tell your doctor or nurse if you have pain. Ways to manage

- **Talk about your pain with a doctor, nurse, or pharmacist. Be specific and describe:**
  - Where you feel pain. Is it in one part of your body or all over?
  - What the pain feels like. Is it sharp, dull, or throbbing? Does it come and go, or is it steady?
  - How strong the pain is. Describe it on a scale of 0 to 10.
  - How long the pain lasts. Does it last for a few minutes, an hour, or longer?
  - What makes the pain better or worse. For instance, does an ice pack help? Or does the pain get worse if you move a certain way?
  - Which medicines you take for pain. Do they help? How long do they last? How much do you take? How often?
- **Let your family and friends know about your pain.** They need to know about your pain so they can help you. If you are very tired or in a lot of pain, they can call your doctor or nurse for you. Knowing about your pain can also help them understand why you may be acting differently.
- **Practice pain control**
  - Take your pain medicine on a regular schedule (by the clock) even when you are not in pain. This is very important when you have pain most of the time.
  - Do not skip doses of your pain medicine. Pain is harder to control and manage if you wait until you are in a lot of pain before taking medicine.
  - Try deep breathing, yoga, or other ways to relax. This can help reduce muscle tension, anxiety, and pain.

- Ask to meet with a pain or palliative care specialist. This can be an oncologist, anesthesiologist, neurologist, neurosurgeon, nurse, or pharmacist who will talk with you about ways to control your pain.
- Let your doctor, nurse, or pain specialist know if your pain changes. Your pain can change over the course of your treatment. When this happens, your pain medications may need to be changed.

NCI's book, *Pain Control: Support for People With Cancer*, provides more tips about how to control pain from cancer and its treatment. You can get free copies at http://www.cancer.gov/publications or by calling 1-800-4-CANCER (1-800-422-6237).

Sexual Changes

What They Are and Why They Occur
Some types of chemotherapy can cause sexual changes. These changes are different for women and men.

In women, chemotherapy may damage the ovaries, which can cause changes in hormone levels. Hormone changes can lead to problems like vaginal dryness and early menopause.

In men, chemotherapy can cause changes in hormone levels, decreased blood supply to the penis, or damage to the nerves that control the penis, all of which can lead to **impotence**.

Whether or not you have sexual changes during chemotherapy depends on if you have had these problems before, the type of chemotherapy you are getting, your age, and whether you have any other illnesses. Some problems, such as loss of interest in sex, are likely to improve once chemotherapy is over.

Problems for WOMEN include:

- Symptoms of menopause (for women not yet in menopause). These symptoms include:
  - Hot flashes
  - Vaginal dryness
  - Feeling irritable
  - Irregular or no menstrual periods
- Bladder or vaginal infections

- Vaginal discharge or itching
- Being too tired to have sex or not being interested in having sex
- Feeling too worried, stressed, or depressed to have sex

Problems for MEN include:

- Not being able to reach climax
- Impotence (not being able to get or keep an erection)
- Being too tired to have sex or not being interested in having sex
- Feeling too worried, stressed, or depressed to have sex

Ways to Manage
For WOMEN:
- Talk with your doctor or nurse about:
    - **Sex.** Ask your doctor or nurse if it is okay for you to have sex during chemotherapy. Most women can have sex, but it is a good idea to ask.
    - **Birth control.** It is very important that you not get pregnant while having chemotherapy. Chemotherapy may hurt the fetus, especially in the first 3 months of pregnancy. If you have not yet gone through menopause, talk with your doctor or nurse about birth control and ways to keep from getting pregnant.
    - **Medications.** Talk with your doctor, nurse, or pharmacist about medications that help with sexual problems. These include products to relieve vaginal dryness or a vaginal cream or suppository to reduce the chance of infection.

Talk with your doctor or nurse about ways to relieve vaginal dryness and prevent infection.

- **Wear cotton underwear (cotton underpants and pantyhose with cotton linings).**
- **Do not wear tight pants or shorts.**
- **Use a water-based vaginal lubricant (such as K-Y Jelly® or Astroglide®) when you have sex.**
- **If sex is still painful because of dryness, ask your doctor or nurse about medications to help restore moisture in your vagina.**
- **Cope with hot flashes by:**

- **Dressing in layers,** with an extra sweater or jacket that you can take off.
- **Being active.** This includes walking, riding a bike, or other types of exercise.
- **Reducing stress.** Try yoga, meditation, or other ways to relax.

For MEN:

- **Talk with your doctor or nurse about:**
  - **Sex.** Ask your doctor or nurse if it is okay for you to have sex during chemotherapy. Most men can have sex, but it is a good idea to ask. Also, ask if you should use a condom when you have sex, since traces of chemotherapy may be in your semen.
  - **Birth control.** It is very important that your spouse or partner not get pregnant while you are getting chemotherapy. Chemotherapy can damage your sperm and cause birth defects.

IF you are having sex less oFten, try activities that make you Feel close to each other.

For men AND women:

- **Be open and honest with your spouse or partner.** Talk about your feelings and concerns.
- **Explore new ways to show love.** You and your spouse or partner may want to show your love for each other in new ways while you go through chemotherapy. For instance, if you are having sex less often, you may want to hug and cuddle more, bathe together, give each other massages, or try other activities that make you feel close to each other.
- **Talk with a doctor, nurse, social worker, or counselor.** If you and your spouse or partner are concerned about sexual problems, you may want to talk with someone who can help. This can be a psychiatrist, psychologist, social worker, marriage counselor, sex therapist, or clergy member.

Ways to Learn More
American Cancer Society
Offers a variety of services to people with cancer and their families.

Call: 1-800-ACS-2345 (1-800-227-2345)
TTY: 1-866-228-4327
Visit: http://www.cancer

Skin and Nail Changes

What They Are and Why They Occur

Some types of chemotherapy can damage the fast-growing cells in your skin and nails. While these changes may be painful and annoying, most are minor and do not require treatment. Many of them will get better once you have finished chemotherapy. However, major skin changes need to be treated right away because they can cause lifelong damage.

Minor skin changes may include:

- **Itching, dryness, redness, rashes, and peeling**
- **Darker veins.** Your veins may look darker when you get chemotherapy through an IV.
- **Sensitivity to the sun** (when you burn very quickly). This can happen even to people who have very dark skin color.
- **Nail problems.** This is when your nails become dark, turn yellow, or become brittle and cracked. Sometimes your nails will loosen and fall off, but new nails will grow back in.

Major skin changes need to be treated right away, because they can cause lifelong changes.

Major skin changes can be caused by:

- **Radiation recall.** Some chemotherapy causes skin in the area where you had radiation therapy to turn red (ranging from very light to bright red). Your skin may blister, peel, or be very painful.
- **Chemotherapy leaking from your IV.** You need to let your doctor or nurse know right away if you have burning or pain when you get IV chemotherapy.
- **Allergic reactions to chemotherapy.** Some skin changes mean that you are allergic to the chemotherapy. Let your doctor or nurse know

right away if you have sudden and severe itching, rashes, or hives, along with wheezing or other trouble breathing.

Let your doctor or nurse know right away if you have burning or pain when you get IV chemotherapy.

Ways to Manage
- **Itching, dryness, redness, rashes, and peeling**
  - Apply cornstarch, as you would dusting powder.
  - Take quick showers or sponge baths instead of long, hot baths.
  - Pat (do not rub) yourself dry after bathing.
  - Wash with a mild, moisturizing soap.
  - Put on cream or lotion while your skin is still damp after washing. Tell your doctor or nurse if this does not help.
  - Do not use perfume, cologne, or aftershave lotion that has alcohol.
  - Take a colloidal oatmeal bath (special powder you add to bath water) when your whole body itches.
- **Acne**
  - Keep your face clean and dry.
  - Ask your doctor or nurse if you can use medicated creams or soaps and which ones to use.
- **Sensitivity to the sun**
  - Avoid direct sunlight. This means not being in the sun from 10 a.m. until 4 p.m. It is the time when the sun is strongest.
  - Use sunscreen lotion with an SPF (skin protection factor) of 15 or higher. Or use ointments that block the sun's rays, such as those with zinc oxide.
  - Keep your lips moist with a lip balm that has an SPF of 15 or higher.
  - Wear light-colored pants, long-sleeve cotton shirts, and hats with wide brims.
  - Do not use tanning beds.
- **Nail problems**
  - Wear gloves when washing dishes, working in the garden, or cleaning the house.
  - Use products to make your nails stronger. (Stop using these products if they hurt your nails or skin.)
  - Let your doctor or nurse know if your cuticles are red and painful.

- **Radiation recall**
  - Protect the area of your skin that received radiation therapy from the sun.
  - Do not use tanning beds.
  - Place a cool, wet cloth where your skin hurts.
  - Wear clothes that are made of cotton or other soft fabrics. This includes your underwear (bras, underpants, and t-shirts).
  - Let your doctor or nurse know if you think you have radiation recall.

Urinary, Kidney, and Bladder Changes

What They Are and Why They Occur

Some types of chemotherapy damage cells in the kidneys and bladder. Problems may include:

- Burning or pain when you begin to urinate or after you empty your bladder
- Frequent, more urgent need to urinate
- Not being able to urinate
- Not able to control the flow of urine from the bladder (**incontinence**)
- Blood in the urine
- Fever
- Chills
- Urine that is orange, red, green, or dark yellow or has a strong medicine odor

Some kidney and bladder problems will go away after you finish chemotherapy. Other problems can last for the rest of your life.

Drink plenty of fluids if you are getting chemotherapy that can damage the bladder and kidneys.

Ways to Manage

- **Your doctor or nurse will take urine and blood samples to check how well your bladder and kidneys are working.**
- **Drink plenty of fluids.** Fluids will help flush the chemotherapy out of your bladder and kidneys.

- **Limit drinks that contain caffeine** (such as black tea, coffee, and some cola products).
- **Talk with your doctor or nurse if you have any of the problems listed above.**

Other Side Effects

Flu-Like Symptoms

Some types of chemotherapy can make you feel like you have the flu. This is more likely to happen if you get chemotherapy along with biological therapy.

Flu-like symptoms may include:

- Muscle and joint aches
- Headache
- Fatigue
- Nausea
- Fever
- Chills
- Appetite loss

These symptoms may last from 1 to 3 days. An infection or the cancer itself can also cause them. Let your doctor or nurse know if you have any of these symptoms.

Fluid Retention

Fluid retention is a buildup of fluid caused by chemotherapy, hormone changes caused by treatment, or your cancer. It can cause your face, hands, feet, or stomach to feel swollen and puffy. Sometimes fluid builds up around your lungs and heart, causing coughing, shortness of breath, or an irregular heart beat. Fluid can also build up in the lower part of your belly, which can cause bloating.

You and your doctor or nurse can help manage fluid retention by:

- Weighing yourself at the same time each day, using the same scale. Let your doctor or nurse know if you gain weight quickly.
- Avoiding table salt or salty foods.

- Limiting the liquids you drink.
- If you retain a lot of fluid, your doctor may prescribe medicine to get rid of the extra fluid.

Eye Changes

- **Trouble wearing contact lenses.** Some types of chemotherapy can bother your eyes and make wearing contact lenses painful. Ask your doctor or nurse if you can wear contact lenses while getting chemotherapy.
- **Blurry vision.** Some types of chemotherapy can clog your tear ducts, which can cause blurry vision.
- **Watery eyes.** Sometimes, chemotherapy can seep out in your tears, which can cause your eyes to water more than usual.

If your vision gets blurry or your eyes water more than usual, tell your doctor or nurse.

FOODS TO HELP WITH SIDE EFFECTS

Clear Liquids

This list may help if you have:

- Diarrhea
- Urinary, kidney, or bladder changes

Type	Examples
Soups	Bouillon
	Clear, fat-free broth Consommé
Drinks	Clear apple juice
	Clear carbonated beverages
	Fruit-flavored drinks
	Fruit juice, such as cranberry or grape
	Fruit punch
	Sports drinks
	Water
	Weak tea with no caffeine

Type	Examples
Sweets	Fruit ices made without fruit pieces or milk Gelatin Honey Jelly Popsicles

Liquid Foods

This list may help if you:

- Do not feel like eating solid foods
- Have urinary, kidney, or bladder changes

Type	Examples	
Soups	Bouillon Broth Cheese soup Soup that has been strained or put through a blender Soup with pureed potatoes Tomato soup	
Drinks	Carbonated beverages Coffee Eggnog (pasteurized and alcohol free) Fruit drinks Fruit juices Fruit punch Milk (all types)	Milkshakes Smoothies Sports drinks Tea Tomato juice Vegetable juice Water
Fats	Butter Cream Margarine Oil Sour cream	
Sweets	Custard (soft or baked) Frozen yogurt Fruit purees that are watered down Gelatin Honey Ice cream with no chunks (such as nuts or cookie pieces) Ice milk	

(Continued)

Type	Examples
	Jelly Pudding Syrup Yogurt (plain or vanilla)
Replacements and supplements	Instant breakfast drinks Liquid meal replacements

Foods and Drinks That Are High in Calories or Protein

This list may help if you do not feel like eating.

Type	Examples	
Soups	Cream soups Soups with lentils, dried peas, or beans (such as pinto, black, red, or kidney)	
Drinks	Instant breakfast drinks Milkshakes Smoothies Whole milk	
Main meals and other foods	Beef Butter, margarine, or oil added to your food Cheese Chicken Cooked dried peas and beans (such as pinto, black, red, or kidney) Cottage cheese	Cream cheese Croissants Deviled ham Eggs Fish Nuts, seeds, and wheat germ Peanut butter Sour cream
Sweets	Custards (soft or baked) Frozen yogurt Ice cream Muffins Pudding Yogurt (plain or vanilla)	
Replacements and supplements	Liquid meal replacements Powdered milk added to foods such as pudding, milkshakes, and scrambled eggs	

High-Fiber Foods

This list may help if you have constipation.

Type	Examples
Main meals and other foods	Bran muffins Bran or whole-grain cereals Brown or wild rice Cooked dried peas and beans (such as pinto, black, red, or kidney) Whole-wheat bread Whole-wheat pastas
Fruits and vegetables	Dried fruit, such as apricots, dates, prunes, and raisins Fresh fruit, such as apples, blueberries, and grapes Raw or cooked vegetables, such as broccoli, corn, green beans, peas, and spinach
Snacks	Granola Nuts Popcorn Seeds, such as sunflower Trail mix

Low-Fiber Foods

This list may help if you have diarrhea.

Type	Examples
Main meals and other foods	Chicken or turkey (skinless) Cooked refined cereals Cottage cheese Eggs Fish Noodles Potatoes (baked or mashed without the skin) White bread White rice
Fruits and vegetables	Asparagus Bananas

(Continued)

Type	Examples
	Canned fruit, such as peaches, pears, and applesauce Clear fruit juice Vegetable juice
Snacks	Angel food cake Gelatin Saltine crackers Sherbet or sorbet Yogurt (plain or vanilla)

Foods That Are Easy on a Sore Mouth

This list may help if your mouth or throat are sore.

Type	Examples
Main meals and other foods	Baby food Cooked refined cereals Cottage cheese Eggs (soft boiled or scrambled) Macaroni and cheese Mashed potatoes Pureed cooked foods Soups
Sweets	Custards Fruit (pureed or baby food) Gelatin Ice cream Milkshakes Puddings Smoothies Soft fruits (bananas and applesauce) Yogurt (plain or vanilla)

Foods and Drinks That Are Easy on the Stomach

This list may help if you have nausea and vomiting.

Type	Examples
Soups	Clear broth, such as chicken, vegetable, or beef
Drinks	Clear carbonated beverages that have lost their fizz Cranberry or grape juice Fruit-flavored drinks Fruit punch Sports drinks Tea Water
Main meals and other foods	Chicken (broiled or baked without its skin) Cream of rice Instant oatmeal Noodles Potatoes (boiled without skins) Pretzels Saltine crackers White rice White toast
Sweets	Angel food cake Canned fruit, such as applesauce, peaches, and pears Gelatin Popsicles Sherbet or sorbet Yogurt (plain or vanilla)

WAYS TO LEARN MORE

National Cancer Institute (NCI)
Find out more from these free NCI services.
Call: 1-800-4-CANCER (1-800-422-6237)
Visit: http://www.cancer
Chat: http://www.cancer
E-mail: cancergovstaff@mail.nih.gov

American Cancer Society
Offers a variety of services to patients and their families. It also supports research, provides printed materials, and conducts educational programs.
Call: 1-800-ACS-2345 (1-800-227-2345); Visit: http://www.cancer

Cancer Support Community
Dedicated to providing support, education, and hope to people affected by cancer.
Call: 1-888-793-9355 or 202-659-9709
Visit: http://www.cancersupportcommunity.org
E-mail: help@cancersupportcommunity.org

Cancer*Care*, Inc.
Offers free support, information, financial assistance, and practical help to people with cancer and their loved ones.
Call: 1-800-813-HOPE (1-800-813-4673)
Visit: http://www.cancercare.org
E-mail: info@cancercare.org

fertileHOPE
A LIVESTRONG initiative dedicated to providing reproductive information, support, and hope to cancer patients and survivors whose medical treatments present the risk of infertility.
Call: 1-866-965-7205
Visit: http://www.fertilehope.org

National Oral Health Information Clearinghouse
A service of the National Institute of Dental and Craniofacial Research that provides oral health information for special care patients.
Call: 1-866-232-4528
Visit: http://www.nidcr.nih.gov
E-mail: nidcrinfo@mail.nih.gov

WORDS TO KNOW

Acupuncture (AK-yoo-PUNK-cher): The technique of inserting thin needles through the skin at specific points on the body to control nausea, vomiting, and other symptoms.

Adjuvant (AD-joo-vant) **chemotherapy**: Chemotherapy used to kill cancer cells after surgery or radiation therapy.

Alopecia (al-oh-PEE-shuh): The lack or loss of hair from areas of the body where hair is usually found. Alopecia can be a side effect of chemotherapy.

Anemia (a-NEE-mee-a): A problem in which the number of red blood cells is below normal.

Antiemetic (AN-tee-eh-MEH-tik): A drug that prevents or controls nausea and vomiting. Also called antinausea.

Antinausea: A drug that prevents or controls nausea and vomiting. Also called antiemetic.

Biological therapy (by-oh-LAH-jih-kul THAYR-uh-pee): Treatment to stimulate or restore the ability of the immune system to fight cancer, infections, and other diseases. Also used to lessen certain side effects that may be caused by some cancer treatments.

Blood cell count: The number of red blood cells, white blood cells, and platelets in a sample of blood. This is also called a complete blood count (CBC).

Bone marrow: The soft, sponge-like tissue in the center of most bones. It produces white blood cells, red blood cells, and platelets.

Cancer clinical trials: Type of research study that tests how well new medical approaches work in people. These studies test new methods of screening, prevention, diagnosis, or treatment of a disease. Also called a clinical study or research study.

Catheter (KATH-i-ter): A flexible tube through which fluids enter or leave the body.

Chemotherapy (kee-moh-THAYR-uh-pee): Treatment with drugs that kill cancer cells.

Constipation: When bowel movements become less frequent and stools are hard, dry, and difficult to pass.

Diarrhea: Frequent bowel movements that may be soft, loose, or watery.

Dry heaves: When your body tries to vomit even though your stomach is empty.

Fatigue: A problem of extreme tiredness and inability to function due lack of energy.

Healthy cells: Noncancerous cells that function the way they should.

Hormones: Chemicals made by glands in the body. Hormones circulate in the bloodstream and control the actions of certain cells or organs.

Impotence: Not being able to get or keep an erection.

Incontinence: Not able to control the flow of urine from the bladder.

Infertility: For women, it means that you may not be able to get pregnant. For men, it means that you may not be able to get a woman pregnant.

Injection: Using a syringe and needle to push fluids or drugs into the body; often called a "shot."

Intra-arterial (IN-truh-ar-TEER-ee-ul): Within an artery. Also called IA.

Intraperitoneal (IN-truh-PAYR-ih-toh-NEE-ul): Within the peritoneal cavity. Also called IP.

Intravenous (in-tra-VEE-nus): Within a blood vessel. Also called IV.

Long-term side effects: Problems from chemotherapy that do not go away.

Metastatic (MET-uh-STAT-ik): The spread of cancer from one part of the body to another. **Nausea**: When you have an upset stomach or queasy feeling and feel like you are going to throw up.

Neo-adjuvant   (NEE-o-AD-joo-vant)   **chemotherapy**:   When chemotherapy is used to shrink a tumor before surgery or radiation therapy.

Neutropenia: An abnormal decrease in the number of neutrophils, a type of white blood cell.

Neutrophil (NOO-tro-fil): A type of white blood cell.

Outpatient: A patient who visits a health care facility for diagnosis or treatment without spending the night.

Palliative (PAL-ee-yuh-tiv) **care**: Care given to improve the quality of life of patients with serious or life-threatening diseases.

Peritoneal (PAYR-ih-toh-NEE-ul) **cavity**: The space within the abdomen that contains the intestines, stomach, liver, ovaries, and other organs.

Platelet (PLATE-let): A type of blood cell that helps prevent bleeding by causing blood clots to form.

Port: An implanted device through which blood may be drawn and drugs may be given without repeated needle sticks.

Pump: A device that is used to deliver a precise amount of a drug at a specific rate.

Radiation therapy: The use of high-energy radiation to kill cancer cells and shrink tumors.

Recurrent: Cancer that returns after not being detected for a period of time.

Red blood cells: Cells that carry oxygen to all parts of the body. Also called RBC.

Side effect: A problem that occurs when treatment affects healthy tissues or organs.

Standard treatment: Treatment that experts agree is appropriate, accepted, and widely used.

Thrombocytopenia (THROM-boh-sy-toh-PEE-nee-uh): A decrease in the number of platelets in the blood that may result in easy bruising and excessive bleeding from wounds or bleeding in mucous membranes and other tissues.

Vomiting: When you throw up.

White blood cells: Cells that help the body fight infection and other diseases. Also called WBC.

In: Cancer Treatment
Editor: Anne E. Wilt

ISBN: 978-1-63321-037-0
© 2014 Nova Science Publishers, Inc.

Chapter 2

RADIATION THERAPY AND YOU: SUPPORT FOR PEOPLE WITH CANCER[*]

National Cancer Institute

ABOUT THIS CHAPTER

Radiation Therapy and You is written for you—someone who is about to get or is now getting radiation therapy for cancer. People who are close to you may also find this chapter helpful.

This chapter is a guide that you can refer to throughout radiation therapy. It has facts about radiation therapy and side effects and describes how you can care for yourself during and after treatment.

This chapter covers:

- **Questions and Answers About Radiation Therapy.** Answers to common questions, such as what radiation therapy is and how it affects cancer cells.
- **External Beam and Internal Radiation.** Information about the two types of radiation therapy.

---

[*] This is an edited, reformatted and augmented version of National Institutes of Health Publication No. 12-7157, revised May 2007.

- **Your Feelings During Radiation Therapy.** Information about feelings, such as depression and anxiety, and ways to cope with them.
- **Side Effects and Ways To Manage Them.** A chart that shows problems that may happen as a result of treatment and ways you can help manage them.
- **Questions To Ask.** Questions for you to think about and discuss with your doctor, nurse, and others involved in your treatment and care.
- **Lists of Foods and Liquids.** Foods and drinks you can have during radiation therapy.
- **Words To Know.** A dictionary that clearly explains medical terms used in this chapter. These terms are in bold print the first time they appear.
- **Ways To Learn More.** Places to go for more information—in print, online (Internet), and by telephone.

Talk with your doctor and nurse about the information in this chapter. They may suggest that you read certain sections or follow some of the tips. Since radiation therapy affects people in different ways, they may also tell you that some of the information in this chapter is not right for you.

QUESTIONS AND ANSWERS ABOUT RADIATION THERAPY

What Is Radiation Therapy?

Radiation therapy (also called radiotherapy) is a cancer treatment that uses high doses of radiation to kill cancer cells and stop them from spreading. At low doses, radiation is used as an x-ray to see inside your body and take pictures, such as x-rays of your teeth or broken bones. Radiation used in cancer treatment works in much the same way, except that it is given at higher doses.

How Is Radiation Therapy Given?

Radiation therapy can be external beam (when a machine outside your body aims radiation at cancer cells) or internal (when radiation is put inside your body, in or near the cancer cells). Sometimes people get both forms of radiation therapy.

Who Gets Radiation Therapy?

Many people with cancer need radiation therapy. In fact, more than half (about 60 percent) of people with cancer get radiation therapy. Sometimes, radiation therapy is the only kind of cancer treatment people need.

What Does Radiation Therapy Do to Cancer Cells?

Given in high doses, radiation kills or slows the growth of cancer cells. Radiation therapy is used to:

- **Treat cancer.** Radiation can be used to cure, stop, or slow the growth of cancer.
- **Reduce symptoms.** When a cure is not possible, radiation may be used to shrink cancer tumors in order to reduce pressure. Radiation therapy used in this way can treat problems such as pain, or it can prevent problems such as blindness or loss of bowel and bladder control.

How Long Does Radiation Therapy Take to Work?

Radiation therapy does not kill cancer cells right away. It takes days or weeks of treatment before cancer cells start to die. Then, cancer cells keep dying for weeks or months after radiation therapy ends.

What Does Radiation Therapy Do to Healthy Cells?

Radiation not only kills or slows the growth of cancer cells, it can also affect nearby healthy cells. The healthy cells almost always recover after treatment is over. But sometimes people may have side effects that do not get better or are severe. Doctors try to protect healthy cells during treatment by:

- **Using as low a dose of radiation as possible.** The radiation dose is balanced between being high enough to kill cancer cells yet low enough to limit damage to healthy cells.

- **Spreading out treatment over time.** You may get radiation therapy once a day for several weeks or in smaller doses twice a day. Spreading out the radiation dose allows normal cells to recover while cancer cells die.
- **Aiming radiation at a precise part of your body.** New techniques, such as **IMRT** and **3-D conformal radiation therapy,** allow your doctor to aim higher doses of radiation at your cancer while reducing the radiation to nearby healthy tissue.
- **Using medicines.** Some drugs can help protect certain parts of your body, such as the salivary glands that make saliva (spit).

Does Radiation Therapy Hurt?

No, radiation therapy does not hurt while it is being given. But the side effects that people may get from radiation therapy can cause pain or discomfort. This chapter has a lot of information about ways that you, your doctor, and your nurse can help manage side effects.

Is Radiation Therapy Used with Other Types of Cancer Treatment?

Yes, radiation therapy is often used with other cancer treatments. Here are some examples:

- **Radiation therapy and surgery.** Radiation may be given before, during, or after surgery. Doctors may use radiation to shrink the size of the cancer before surgery, or they may use radiation after surgery to kill any cancer cells that remain. Sometimes, radiation therapy is given during surgery so that it goes straight to the cancer without passing through the skin. This is called intraoperative radiation.
- **Radiation therapy and chemotherapy.** Radiation may be given before, during, or after chemotherapy. Before or during chemotherapy, radiation therapy can shrink the cancer so that chemotherapy works better. Sometimes, chemotherapy is given to help radiation therapy work better. After chemotherapy, radiation therapy can be used to kill any cancer cells that remain.

Who Is on My Radiation Therapy Team?

Many people help with your radiation treatment and care. This group of health care providers is often called the "radiation therapy team." They work together to provide care that is just right for you. Your radiation therapy team can include:

- **Radiation oncologist.** This is a doctor who specializes in using radiation therapy to treat cancer. He or she prescribes how much radiation you will receive, plans how your treatment will be given, closely follows you during your course of treatment, and prescribes care you may need to help with side effects. He or she works closely with the other doctors, nurses, and health care providers on your team. After you are finished with radiation therapy, your radiation oncologist will see you for follow-up visits. During these visits, this doctor will check for **late side effects** and assess how well the radiation has worked.
- **Nurse practitioner.** This is a nurse with advanced training. He or she can take your medical history, do physical exams, order tests, manage side effects, and closely watch your response to treatment. After you are finished with radiation therapy, your nurse practitioner may see you for follow-up visits to check for late side effects and assess how well the radiation has worked.
- **Radiation nurse.** This person provides nursing care during radiation therapy, working with all the members of your radiation therapy team. He or she will talk with you about your radiation treatment and help you manage side effects.
- **Radiation therapist.** This person works with you during each radiation therapy session. He or she positions you for treatment and runs the machines to make sure you get the dose of radiation prescribed by your radiation oncologist.
- **Other health care providers.** Your team may also include a dietitian, physical therapist, social worker, and others.
- **You.** You are also part of the radiation therapy team. Your role is to:
  - Arrive on time for all radiation therapy sessions
  - Ask questions and talk about your concerns
  - Let someone on your radiation therapy team know when you have side effects
  - Tell your doctor or nurse if you are in pain

- Follow the advice of your doctors and nurses about how to care for yourself at home, such as:
  - Taking care of your skin
  - Drinking liquids
  - Eating foods that they suggest - Keeping your weight the same

Is Radiation Therapy Expensive?

Yes, radiation therapy costs a lot of money. It uses complex machines and involves the services of many health care providers. The exact cost of your radiation therapy depends on the cost of health care where you live, what kind of radiation therapy you get, and how many treatments you need.

Talk with your health insurance company about what services it will pay for. Most insurance plans pay for radiation therapy for their members. To learn more, talk with the business office where you get treatment. You can also contact the National Cancer Institute's Cancer Information Service and ask for the "Financial Assistance for Cancer Care" fact sheet.

Should I Follow a Special Diet While I Am Getting Radiation Therapy?

Your body uses a lot of energy to heal during radiation therapy. It is important that you eat enough calories and protein to keep your weight the same during this time. Ask your doctor or nurse if you need a special diet while you are getting radiation therapy. You might also find it helpful to speak with a dietitian.

To learn more about foods and drinks that are high in calories or protein, see the chart later in this chapter. You may also want to read Eating Hints, a book from the National Cancer Institute. You can order a free copy online at http://www.cancer.gov/ publications or 1-800-4-CANCER.

Can I Go to Work During Radiation Therapy?

Some people are able to work full-time during radiation therapy. Others can only work part-time or not at all. How much you are able to work depends on how you feel. Ask your doctor or nurse what you may expect based on the treatment you are getting.

You are likely to feel well enough to work when you start radiation therapy. As time goes on, do not be surprised if you are more tired, have less energy, or feel weak. Once you have finished your treatment, it may take a few weeks or many months for you to feel better.

You may get to a point during your radiation therapy when you feel too sick to work. Talk with your employer to find out if you can go on medical leave. Make sure that your health insurance will pay for treatment when you are on medical leave.

What Happens When Radiation Therapy Is over?

Once you have finished radiation therapy, you will need follow-up care for the rest of your life. Follow-up care refers to checkups with your radiation oncologist or nurse practitioner after your course of radiation therapy is over. During these checkups, your doctor or nurse will see how well the radiation therapy worked, check for other signs of cancer, look for late side effects, and talk with you about your treatment and care. Your doctor or nurse will:

- **Examine you and review how you have been feeling.** Your doctor or nurse practitioner can prescribe medicine or suggest other ways to treat any side effects you may have.
- **Order lab and imaging tests.** These may include blood tests, x-rays, or CT, MRI, or PET scans.
- **Discuss treatment.** Your doctor or nurse practitioner may suggest that you have more treatment, such as extra radiation treatments, chemotherapy, or both.
- **Answer your questions and respond to your concerns.** It may be helpful to write down your questions ahead of time and bring them with you. You can find sample questions later in this chapter.

After Radiation Therapy Is over, What Symptoms Should I Look for?

You have gone through a lot with cancer and radiation therapy. Now you may be even more aware of your body and how you feel each day. Pay

attention to changes in your body and let your doctor or nurse know if you
have:

- A pain that does not go away
- New lumps, bumps, swellings, rashes, bruises, or bleeding
- Appetite changes, **nausea**, **vomiting**, diarrhea, or constipation
- Weight loss that you cannot explain
- A fever, cough, or hoarseness that does not go away
- Any other symptoms that worry you

EXTERNAL BEAM RADIATION THERAPY

What Is External Beam Radiation Therapy?

External beam radiation therapy comes from a machine that aims radiation
at your cancer. The machine is large and may be noisy. It does not touch you,
but rotates around you, sending radiation to your body from many directions.

External beam radiation therapy is a **local treatment**, meaning that the
radiation is aimed only at a specific part of your body. For example, if you
have lung cancer, you will get radiation to your chest only and not the rest of
your body.

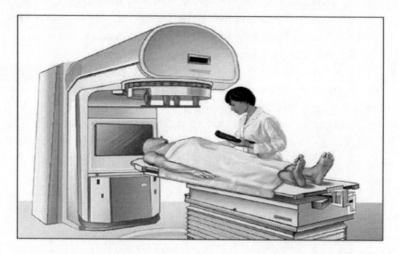

External beam radiation therapy comes from a machine that aims radiation at your
cancer.

How Often Will I Get External Beam Radiation Therapy?

Most people get external beam radiation therapy once a day, 5 days a week, Monday through Friday. Treatment lasts for 2 to 10 weeks, depending on the type of cancer you have and the goal of your treatment. The time between your first and last radiation therapy sessions is called a course of treatment.

Radiation is sometimes given in smaller doses twice a day (hyperfractionated radiation therapy). Your doctor may prescribe this type of treatment if he or she feels that it will work better. Although side effects may be more severe, there may be fewer late side effects. Doctors are doing research to see which types of cancer are best treated this way.

Where Do I Go for External Beam Radiation Therapy?

Most of the time, you will get external beam radiation therapy as an outpatient. This means that you will have treatment at a clinic or radiation therapy center and will not have to stay in the hospital.

What Happens Before My First External Beam Radiation Treatment?

You will have a 1- to 2-hour meeting with your doctor or nurse before you begin radiation therapy. At this time, you will have a physical exam, talk about your medical history, and maybe have imaging tests. Your doctor or nurse will discuss external beam radiation therapy, its benefits and side effects, and ways you can care for yourself during and after treatment. You can then choose whether to have external beam radiation therapy.

If you agree to have external beam radiation therapy, you will be scheduled for a treatment planning session called a **simulation**. At this time:

- A radiation oncologist and radiation therapist will define your treatment area (also called a **treatment port** or **treatment field**). This refers to the places in your body that will get radiation. You will be asked to lie very still while x-rays or scans are taken to define the treatment area.

- The radiation therapist will then put small marks (tattoos or dots of colored ink) on your skin to mark the treatment area. You will need these marks throughout the course of radiation therapy. The radiation therapist will use them each day to make sure you are in the correct position. Tattoos are about the size of a freckle and will remain on your skin for the rest of your life. Ink markings will fade over time. Be careful not to remove them and make sure to tell the radiation therapist if they fade or lose color.

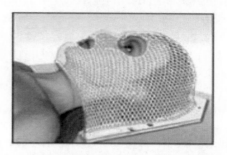

If you are getting radiation to the head, you may need a mask.

- You may need a body mold. This is a plastic or plaster form that helps keep you from moving during treatment. It also helps make sure that you are in the exact same position each day of treatment.
- If you are getting radiation to the head, you may need a mask. The mask has air holes, and holes can be cut for your eyes, nose, and mouth. It attaches to the table where you will lie to receive your treatments. The mask helps keep your head from moving so that you are in the exact same position for each treatment.

What Should I Wear When I Get External Beam Radiation Therapy?

Wear clothes that are comfortable and made of soft fabric, such as cotton. Choose clothes that are easy to take off, since you may need to change into a hospital gown or show the area that is being treated. Do not wear clothes that are tight, such as close-fitting collars or waistbands, near your treatment area. Also, do not wear jewelry, BAND-AIDS®, powder, lotion, or deodorant in or near your treatment area, and do not use deodorant soap before your treatment.

What Happens during Treatment Sessions?

- You may be asked to change into a hospital gown or robe.
- You will go to a treatment room where you will receive radiation.
- Depending on where your cancer is, you will either sit in a chair or lie down on a treatment table. The radiation therapist will use your body mold and skin marks to help you get into position.
- You may see colored lights pointed at your skin marks. These lights are harmless and help the therapist position you for treatment each day.
- You will need to stay very still so the radiation goes to the exact same place each time. You can breathe as you always do and do not have to hold your breath.

The radiation therapist will leave the room just before your treatment begins. He or she will go to a nearby room to control the radiation machine and watch you on a TV screen or through a window. You are not alone, even though it may feel that way. The radiation therapist can see you on the screen or through the window. He or she can hear and talk with you through a speaker in your treatment room. Make sure to tell the therapist if you feel sick or are uncomfortable. He or she can stop the radiation machine at any time. You cannot feel, hear, see, or smell radiation.

Your entire visit may last from 30 minutes to 1 hour. Most of that time is spent setting you in the correct position. You will get radiation for only 1 to 5 minutes. If you are getting IMRT, your treatment may last longer. Your visit may also take longer if your treatment team needs to take and review x-rays.

Will External Beam Radiation Therapy Make Me Radioactive?

No, external beam radiation therapy does not make people radioactive. You may safely be around other people, even babies and young children.

How Can I Relax during My Treatment Sessions?

Bring something to read or do while in the waiting room.

- Ask if you can listen to music or books on tape.

- Meditate, breathe deeply, use imagery, or find other ways to relax. To learn more about ways to relax, see *Facing Forward: Life After Cancer Treatment*, a book from the National Cancer Institute. You can order a free copy at http://www.cancer or 1-800-4-CANCER.

INTERNAL RADIATION THERAPY

What Is Internal Radiation Therapy?

Internal radiation therapy is a form of treatment where a source of radiation is put inside your body. One form of internal radiation therapy is called brachytherapy. In brachytherapy, the radiation source is a solid in the form of seeds, ribbons, or capsules, which are placed in your body in or near the cancer cells. This allows treatment with a high dose of radiation to a smaller part of your body. Internal radiation can also be in a liquid form. You receive liquid radiation by drinking it, by swallowing a pill, or through an IV. Liquid radiation travels throughout your body, seeking out and killing cancer cells.

Brachytherapy may be used with people who have cancers of the head, neck, breast, uterus, cervix, prostate, gall bladder, esophagus, eye, and lung. Liquid forms of internal radiation are most often used with people who have thyroid cancer or non-Hodgkin's lymphoma. You may also get internal radiation along with other types of treatment, including external beam radiation, chemotherapy, or surgery.

What Happens Before My First Internal Radiation Treatment?

You will have a 1- to 2-hour meeting with your doctor or nurse before you begin internal radiation therapy. At this time, you will have a physical exam, talk about your medical history, and maybe have imaging tests. Your doctor will discuss the type of internal radiation therapy that is best for you, its benefits and side effects, and ways you can care for yourself during and after treatment. You can then choose whether to have internal radiation therapy.

How Is Brachytherapy Put in Place?

Most brachytherapy is put in place through a catheter, which is a small, stretchy tube. Sometimes, it is put in place through a larger device called an applicator. When you decide to have brachytherapy, your doctor will place the catheter or applicator into the part of your body that will be treated.

What Happens When the Catheter or Applicator Is Put in Place?

You will most likely be in the hospital when your catheter or applicator is put in place. Here is what to expect:

- You will either be put to sleep or the area where the catheter or applicator goes will be numbed. This will help prevent pain when it is put in.
- Your doctor will place the catheter or applicator in your body.
- If you are awake, you may be asked to lie very still while the catheter or applicator is put in place. If you feel any discomfort, tell your doctor or nurse so he or she can give you medicine to help manage the pain.

What Happens after the Catheter or Applicator Is Placed in My Body?

Once your treatment plan is complete, radiation will be placed inside the catheter or applicator. The radiation source may be kept in place for a few minutes, many days, or the rest of your life. How long the radiation is in place depends on which type of brachytherapy you get, your type of cancer, where the cancer is in your body, your health, and other cancer treatments you have had.

What Are the Types of Brachytherapy?

There are three types of brachytherapy:

- **Low-dose rate (LDR) implants.** In this type of brachytherapy, radiation stays in place for 1 to 7 days. You are likely to be in the hospital during this time. Once your treatment is finished, your doctor will remove the radiation sources and your catheter or applicator.
- **High-dose rate (HDR) implants.** In this type of brachytherapy, the radiation source is in place for 10 to 20 minutes at a time and then taken out. You may have treatment twice a day for 2 to 5 days or once a week for 2 to 5 weeks. The schedule depends on your type of cancer. During the course of treatment, your catheter or applicator may stay in place, or it may be put in place before each treatment. You may be in the hospital during this time, or you may make daily trips to the hospital to have the radiation source put in place. Like LDR implants, your doctor will remove your catheter or applicator once you have finished treatment.
- **Permanent implants.** After the radiation source is put in place, the catheter is removed. The implants always stay in your body, while the radiation gets weaker each day. You may need to limit your time around other people when the radiation is first put in place. Be extra careful not to spend time with children or pregnant women. As time goes by, almost all the radiation will go away, even though the implant stays in your body.

What Happens While the Radiation Is in Place?

- Your body will give off radiation once the radiation source is in place. With brachytherapy, your body fluids (urine, sweat, and saliva) will not give off radiation. With liquid radiation, your body fluids will give off radiation for a while.
- Your doctor or nurse will talk with you about safety measures that you need to take.
- If the radiation you receive is a very high dose, safety measures may include:
  - Staying in a private hospital room to protect others from radiation coming from your body
  - Being treated quickly by nurses and other hospital staff. They will provide all the care you need, but they may stand at a distance and talk with you from the doorway to your room.

- Your visitors will also need to follow safety measures, which may include:
    - Not being allowed to visit when the radiation is first put in
    - Needing to check with the hospital staff before they go to your room
    - Keeping visits short (30 minutes or less each day). The length of visits depends on the type of radiation being used and the part of your body being treated.
    - Standing by the doorway rather than going into your hospital room
    - Not having visits from children younger than 18 and pregnant women

You may also need to follow safety measures once you leave the hospital, such as not spending much time with other people. Your doctor or nurse will talk with you about the safety measures you should follow when you go home.

What Happens When the Catheter Is Taken out after Treatment With LDR or HDR Implants?

- You will get medicine for pain before the catheter or applicator is removed.
- The area where the catheter or applicator was might be tender for a few months.
- There is no radiation in your body after the catheter or applicator is removed. It is safe for people to be near you— even young children and pregnant women.
- For 1 to 2 weeks, you may need to limit activities that take a lot of effort. Ask your doctor what kinds of activities are safe for you.

YOUR FEELINGS DURING RADIATION THERAPY

At some point during radiation therapy, you may feel:

- Anxious
- Depressed
- Afraid

- Angry
- Frustrated
- Helpless
- Alone

It is normal to have these kinds of feelings. Living with cancer and going through treatment is stressful. You may also feel **fatigue**, which can make it harder to cope with these feelings.

How Can I Cope with My Feelings during Radiation Therapy?

There are many things you can do to cope with your feelings during treatment. Here are some things that have worked for other people:

- **Relax and meditate.** You might try thinking of yourself in a favorite place, breathing slowly while paying attention to each breath, or listening to soothing music. These kinds of activities can help you feel calmer and less stressed.
- **Exercise.** Many people find that light exercise (such as walking, biking, yoga, or water aerobics) helps them feel better. Talk with your doctor or nurse about types of exercise that you can do.
- **Talk with others.** Talk about your feelings with someone you trust. You may choose a close friend, family member, chaplain, nurse, social worker, or psychologist. You may also find it helpful to talk to someone else who is going through radiation therapy.
- **Join a support group.** Cancer **support groups** are meetings for people with cancer. These groups allow you to meet others facing the same problems. You will have a chance to talk about your feelings and listen to other people talk about theirs. You can learn how others cope with cancer, radiation therapy, and side effects. Your doctor, nurse, or social worker can tell you about support groups near where you live. Some support groups also meet over the Internet, which can be helpful if you cannot travel or find a meeting in your area.
- **Talk to your doctor or nurse about things that worry or upset you.** You may want to ask about seeing a counselor. Your doctor may also suggest that you take medicine if you find it very hard to cope with these feelings.

Ways to Learn More

To learn more about ways to cope with your feelings, read *Taking Time: Support for People with Cancer*, a book from the National Cancer Institute. You can get a free copy at http://www.cancer or 1-800-4-CANCER (1-800-422-6237).

CancerCare, Inc.
Offers free support, information, financial assistance, and practical help to people with cancer and their loved ones.
Toll-free: 1-800-813-HOPE (1-800-813-4673)
E-mail: info@cancercare.org
Online: http://www.cancercare.org

The Wellness Community
Provides free psychological and emotional support to people with cancer and their families.
Toll-free: 1-888-793-WELL (1-888-793-9355)
Phone: 202-659-9709
Online: http://www.thewellnesscommunity.org
E-mail: help@thewellnesscommunity.org

RADIATION THERAPY SIDE EFFECTS

Side effects are problems that can happen as a result of treatment. They may happen with radiation therapy because the high doses of radiation used to kill cancer cells can also damage healthy cells in the treatment area. Side effects are different for each person. Some people have many side effects; others have hardly any. Side effects may be more severe if you also receive chemotherapy before, during, or after your radiation therapy.

Talk to your radiation therapy team about your chances of having side effects. The team will watch you closely and ask if you notice any problems. If you do have side effects or other problems, your doctor or nurse will talk with you about ways to manage them.

Common Side Effects
Many people who get radiation therapy have skin changes and some fatigue. Other side effects depend on the part of your body being treated.

Skin changes may include dryness, itching, peeling, or blistering. These changes occur because radiation therapy damages healthy skin cells in the treatment area. You will need to take special care of your skin during radiation therapy.

Fatigue is often described as feeling worn out or exhausted. There are many ways to manage fatigue.

Depending on the part of your body being treated, you may also have:

- Diarrhea
- Hair loss in treatment area
- Mouth problems
- Nausea and vomiting
- Sexual changes
- Swelling
- Trouble swallowing
- Urinary and bladder changes

Most of these side effects go away within 2 months after radiation therapy is finished.

Late side effects may first occur 6 or more months after radiation therapy is over. They vary by the part of your body that was treated and the dose of radiation you received. Late side effects may include **infertility**, joint problems, lymphedema, mouth problems, and secondary cancer. Everyone is different, so talk to your doctor or nurse about whether you might have late side effects and what signs to look for.

Radiation Therapy Side Effects and Ways To Manage Them, explains each side effect in more detail and includes ways you and your doctor or nurse can help manage them.

Radiation Therapy Side Effects at-a-Glance

Radiation therapy side effects depend on the part of your body being treated. You can use the chart to see which side effects might affect you. Find the part of your body being treated in the column on the left, then read across the row to see the side effects. A checkmark means that you may get this side effect. Ask your doctor or nurse about your chances of getting each side effect.

	Diarrhea	Fatigue	Hair Loss (on the part of the body being treated)	Mouth Changes	Nausea and Vomiting	Sexual and Fertility Changes	Skin Changes	Throat Changes	Urinary and Bladder Changes	Other Side Effects
Brain		✓	✓		✓		✓			Headache Blurry vision
Breast		✓	✓				✓			Tenderness Swelling
Chest		✓	✓				✓	✓		Cough Shortness of breath
Head and Neck		✓	✓	✓			✓	✓		Earaches Taste changes
Pelvic Area	✓	✓	✓		✓	✓	✓		✓	
Rectum	✓	✓	✓			✓	✓		✓	
Stomach and Abdomen	✓	✓	✓		✓		✓		✓	

Radiation Therapy Side Effects at-a-Glance

- Find the part of your body being treated in the column on the left.
- Read across the row.
- A checkmark means you may get the side effect listed.

Radiation Therapy Side Effects and Ways to Manage Them

Diarrhea

What It Is
Diarrhea is frequent bowel movements which may be soft, formed, loose, or watery. Diarrhea can occur at any time during radiation therapy.

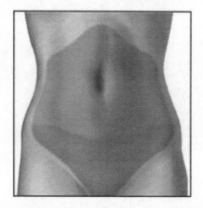

Radiation to the shaded area may cause diarrhea.

Why It Occurs
Radiation therapy to the pelvis, stomach, and abdomen can cause diarrhea. People get diarrhea because radiation harms the healthy cells in the large and small bowels. These areas are very sensitive to the amount of radiation needed to treat cancer.

Ways to Manage
When you have diarrhea:

- **Drink 8 to 12 cups of clear liquid per day.**

If you drink liquids that are high in sugar (such as fruit juice, sweet iced tea, Kool-Aid®, or Hi-C®) ask your nurse or dietitian if you should mix them with water.

- **Eat many small meals and snacks.** For instance, eat 5 or 6 small meals and snacks rather than 3 large meals.

- **Eat foods that are easy on the stomach (which means foods that are low in fiber, fat, and lactose).** If your diarrhea is severe, your doctor or nurse may suggest the BRAT diet, which stands for bananas, rice, applesauce, and toast.

- **Take care of your rectal area.** Instead of toilet paper, use a baby wipe or squirt of water from a spray bottle to clean yourself after bowel movements. Also, ask your nurse about taking sitz baths, which is a warm-water bath taken in a sitting position that covers only the hips and buttocks. Be sure to tell your doctor or nurse if your rectal area gets sore.

- **Stay away from:**
  - Milk and dairy foods, such as ice cream, sour cream, and cheese
  - Spicy foods, such as hot sauce, salsa, chili, and curry dishes
  - Foods or drinks with caffeine, such as regular coffee, black tea, soda, and chocolate
  - Foods or drinks that cause gas, such as cooked dried beans, cabbage, broccoli, soy milk, and other soy products
  - Foods that are high in fiber, such as raw fruits and vegetables, cooked dried beans, and whole wheat breads and cereals
  - Fried or greasy foods
  - Food from fast food restaurants

- **Talk to your doctor or nurse.** Tell them if you are having diarrhea. He or she will suggest ways to manage it. He or she may also suggest taking medicine, such as Imodium®.

To learn more about dealing with diarrhea during cancer treatment, see *Eating Hints: Before, During, and After Cancer Treatment*, a book from the National Cancer Institute. You can get a free copy at http://www.cancer.gov/publications or 1-800-4-CANCER (1-800-422-6237).

Fatigue

What It Is

Fatigue from radiation therapy can range from a mild to an extreme feeling of being tired. Many people describe fatigue as feeling weak, weary, worn out, heavy, or slow.

Why It Occurs

Fatigue can happen for many reasons. These include:

- Anemia
- Anxiety
- Depression
- Infection
- Lack of activity
- Medicines

Fatigue can also come from the effort of going to radiation therapy each day or from stress. Most of the time, you will not know why you feel fatigue.

How Long It Lasts

When you first feel fatigue depends on a few factors, which include your age, health, level of activity, and how you felt before radiation therapy started.

Fatigue can last from 6 weeks to 12 months after your last radiation therapy session. Some people may always feel fatigue and, even after radiation therapy is over, will not have as much energy as they did before.

Ways to Manage

- **Try to sleep at least 8 hours each night.** This may be more sleep than you needed before radiation therapy. One way to sleep better at night is to be active during the day. For example, you could go for walks, do yoga, or ride a bike. Another way to sleep better at night is to relax before going to bed. You might read a book, work on a jigsaw puzzle, listen to music, or do other calming hobbies.
- **Plan time to rest.** You may need to nap during the day. Many people say that it helps to rest for just 10 to 15 minutes. If you do nap, try to sleep for less than 1 hour at a time.
- **Try not to do too much.** With fatigue, you may not have enough energy to do all the things you want to do. Stay active, but choose the

activities that are most important to you. For example, you might go to work but not do housework, or watch your children's sports events but not go out to dinner.

- **Exercise.** Most people feel better when they get some exercise each day. Go for a 15- to 30-minute walk or do stretches or yoga. Talk with your doctor or nurse about how much exercise you can do while having radiation therapy.
- **Plan a work schedule that is right for you.** Fatigue may affect the amount of energy you have for your job. You may feel well enough to work your full schedule, or you may need to work less—maybe just a few hours a day or a few days each week. You may want to talk with your boss about ways to work from home so you do not have to commute. And you may want to think about going on medical leave while you have radiation therapy.
- **Plan a radiation therapy schedule that makes sense for you.** You may want to schedule your radiation therapy around your work or family schedule. For example, you might want to have radiation therapy in the morning so you can go to work in the afternoon.
- **Let others help you at home.** Check with your insurance company to see whether it covers home care services. You can also ask family members and friends to help when you feel fatigue. Home care staff, family members, and friends can assist with household chores, running errands, or driving you to and from radiation therapy visits. They might also help by cooking meals for you to eat now or freeze for later.
- **Learn from others who have cancer.** People who have cancer can help each other by sharing ways to manage fatigue. One way to meet other people with cancer is by joining a support group—either in person or online. Talk with your doctor or nurse to learn more about support groups.
- **Talk with your doctor or nurse.** If you have trouble dealing with fatigue, your doctor may prescribe medicine (called **psychostimulants**) that can help decrease fatigue, give you a sense of well-being, and increase your appetite. Your doctor may also suggest treatments if you have anemia, depression, or are not able to sleep at night.

Hair Loss

What It Is
Hair loss (also called **alopecia**) is when some or all of your hair falls out.

Why It Occurs
Radiation therapy can cause hair loss because it damages cells that grow quickly, such as those in your hair roots.

Hair loss from radiation therapy only happens on the part of your body being treated. This is not the same as hair loss from chemotherapy, which happens all over your body. For instance, you may lose some or all of the hair on your head when you get radiation to your brain. But if you get radiation to your hip, you may lose pubic hair (between your legs) but not the hair on your head.

How Long It Lasts
You may start losing hair in your treatment area 2 to 3 weeks after your first radiation therapy session. It takes about a week for all the hair in your treatment area to fall out. Your hair may grow back 3 to 6 months after treatment is over. Sometimes, though, the dose of radiation is so high that your hair never grows back.

Once your hair starts to grow back, it may not look or feel the way it did before. Your hair may be thinner, or curly instead of straight. Or it may be darker or lighter in color than it was before.

Ways to Manage Hair Loss on Your Head

Before hair loss:

- **Decide whether to cut your hair or shave your head.** You may feel more in control of hair loss when you plan ahead. Use an electric razor to prevent nicking yourself if you decide to shave your head.
- **If you plan to buy a wig, do so while you still have hair.** The best time to select your wig is before radiation therapy begins or soon after it starts. This way, the wig will match the color and style of your own hair. Some people take their wig to their hair stylist. You will want to have your wig fitted once you have lost your hair. Make sure to choose a wig that feels comfortable and does not hurt your scalp.

- **Check with your health insurance company to see whether it will pay for your wig.** If it does not, you can deduct the cost of your wig as a medical expense on your income taxes. Some groups also sponsor free wig banks. Ask your doctor, nurse, or social worker if he or she can refer you to a free wig bank in your area.
- **Be gentle when you wash your hair.** Use a mild shampoo, such as a baby shampoo. Dry your hair by patting (not rubbing) it with a soft towel.
- **Do not use curling irons, electric hair dryers, curlers, hair bands, clips, or hair sprays.** These can hurt your scalp or cause early hair loss.
- **Do not use products that are harsh on your hair.** These include hair colors, perms, gels, mousse, oil, grease, or pomade.

After hair loss:

- **Protect your scalp.** Your scalp may feel tender after hair loss. Cover your head with a hat, turban, or scarf when you are outside. Try not to be in places where the temperature is very cold or very hot. This means staying away from the direct sun, sun lamps, and very cold air.
- **Stay warm.** Your hair helps keep you warm, so you may feel colder once you lose it. You can stay warmer by wearing a hat, turban, scarf, or wig.

Ways to Learn More

American Cancer Society
Offers a variety of services to people with cancer and their families, including referrals to low-cost wig banks.
Toll-free: 1-800-ACS-2345 (1-800-227-2345)
Phone: 404-320-3333
Online: http://www.cancer

Mouth Changes

What They Are
Radiation therapy to the head or neck can cause problems such as:

- Mouth sores (little cuts or ulcers in your mouth)

- Dry mouth (also called **xerostomia**) and throat
- Loss of taste
- Tooth decay
- Changes in taste (such as a metallic taste when you eat meat)
- Infections of your gums, teeth, or tongue
- Jaw stiffness and bone changes
- Thick, rope-like saliva

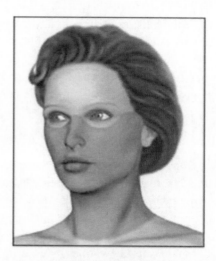

Radiation to the shaded area may cause mouth changes.

Why They Occur

Radiation therapy kills cancer cells and can also damage healthy cells such as those in the glands that make saliva and the soft, moist lining of your mouth.

How Long They Last

Some problems, like mouth sores, may go away after treatment ends. Others, such as taste changes, may last for months or even years. Some problems, like dry mouth, may never go away.

Ways to Manage

- If you are getting radiation therapy to your head or neck, **visit a dentist at least 2 weeks before treatment starts.** At this time, your dentist will examine your teeth and mouth and do any needed dental work to make sure your mouth is as healthy as possible before radiation therapy. If you cannot get to the dentist before treatment starts, ask your doctor if you should schedule a visit soon after treatment begins.

- **Check your mouth every day.** This way, you can see or feel problems as soon as they start. Problems can include mouth sores, white patches, or infection.
- **Keep your mouth moist.** You can do this by:
  - Sipping water often during the day
  - Sucking on ice chips
  - Chewing sugar-free gum or sucking on sugar-free hard candy
  - Using a saliva substitute to help moisten your mouth
  - Asking your doctor to prescribe medicine that helps increase saliva
- **Clean your mouth, teeth, gums, and tongue.**
  - Brush your teeth, gums, and tongue after every meal and at bedtime.
  - Use an extra-soft toothbrush. You can make the bristles softer by running warm water over them just before you brush.
  - Use a fluoride toothpaste.
  - Use a special fluoride gel that your dentist can prescribe.
  - Do not use mouthwashes that contain alcohol.
  - Gently floss your teeth every day. If your gums bleed or hurt, avoid those areas but floss your other teeth.
  - Rinse your mouth every 1 to 2 hours with a solution of 1/4 teaspoon baking soda and 1/8 teaspoon salt mixed in 1 cup of warm water.
  - If you have dentures, make sure they fit well and limit how long you wear them each day. If you lose weight, your dentist may need to adjust them.
  - Keep your dentures clean by soaking or brushing them each day.
- **Be careful what you eat when your mouth is sore.**
  - Choose foods that are easy to chew and swallow.
  - Take small bites, chew slowly, and sip liquids with your meals.
  - Eat moist, soft foods such as cooked cereals, mashed potatoes, and scrambled eggs.
  - Wet and soften food with gravy, sauce, broth, yogurt, or other liquids.
  - Eat foods that are warm or at room temperature.

- **Stay away from things that can hurt, scrape, or burn your mouth, such as:**
  - Sharp, crunchy foods such as potato or corn chips
  - Hot foods
  - Spicy foods such as hot sauce, curry dishes, salsa, and chili
  - Fruits and juices that are high in acid such as tomatoes, oranges, lemons, and grapefruits
  - Toothpicks or other sharp objects
  - All tobacco products, including cigarettes, pipes, cigars, and chewing tobacco
  - Drinks that contain alcohol
- **Stay away from foods and drinks that are high in sugar.** Foods and drinks that have a lot sugar (such as regular soda, gum, and candy) can cause tooth decay.
- **Exercise your jaw muscles.**
  Open and close your mouth 20 times as far as you can without causing pain. Do this exercise 3 times a day, even if your jaw isn't stiff.

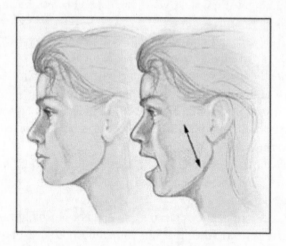

Exercise your jaw 3 times a day.

- **Medicine.** Ask your doctor or nurse about medicines that can protect your saliva glands and the moist tissues that line your mouth.
- **Call your doctor or nurse when your mouth hurts.** There are medicines and other products, such as mouth gels, that can help control mouth pain.

- **You will need to take extra good care of your mouth for the rest of your life.** Ask your dentist how often you will need dental check-ups and how best to take care of your teeth and mouth after radiation therapy is over.

Ways to Learn More

National Oral Health Information Clearinghouse

A service of the National Institute of Dental and Craniofacial Research that provides oral health information for special care patients.

Phone: 301-402-7364

Online: http://www.nidcr.nih.gov

Smokefree.gov

Provides resources, including information on quit lines, a step-by-step cessation guide, and publications, to help you or someone you care about quit smoking.

Toll-free: 1-877-44U-QUIT (1-877-448-7848)

Online: http://www.smokefree.gov

Nausea and Vomiting

What They Are

Radiation therapy can cause nausea, vomiting, or both. Nausea is when you feel sick to your stomach and feel like you are going to throw up. Vomiting is when you throw up food and fluids. You may also have **dry heaves**, which happen when your body tries to vomit even though your stomach is empty.

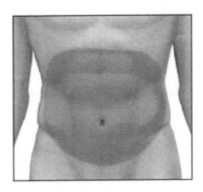

Radiation to the shaded area may cause nausea and vomiting.

Why They Occur

Nausea and vomiting can occur after radiation therapy to the stomach, small intestine, colon, or parts of the brain. Your risk for nausea and vomiting depends on how much radiation you are getting, how much of your body is in the treatment area, and whether you are also having chemotherapy.

How Long They Last

Nausea and vomiting may occur 30 minutes to many hours after your radiation therapy session ends. You are likely to feel better on days that you do not have radiation therapy.

Ways to Manage

- **Prevent nausea.** The best way to keep from vomiting is to prevent nausea. One way to do this is by having bland, easy-to-digest foods and drinks that do not upset your stomach. These include toast, gelatin, and apple juice.
- **Try to relax before treatment.** You may feel less nausea if you relax before each radiation therapy treatment. You can do this by spending time doing activities you enjoy, such as reading a book, listening to music, or other hobbies.
- **Plan when to eat and drink.** Some people feel better when they eat before radiation therapy; others do not. Learn the best time for you to eat and drink. For example, you might want a snack of crackers and apple juice 1 to 2 hours before radiation therapy. Or, you might feel better if you have treatment on an empty stomach, which means not eating 2 to 3 hours before treatment.
- **Eat small meals and snacks.** Instead of eating 3 large meals each day, you may want to eat 5 or 6 small meals and snacks. Make sure to eat slowly and do not rush.
- **Have foods and drinks that are warm or cool (not hot or cold).** Before eating or drinking, let hot food and drinks cool down and cold food and drinks warm up.
- **Talk with your doctor or nurse.** He or she may suggest a special diet of foods to eat or prescribe medicine to help prevent nausea, which you can take 1 hour before each radiation therapy session. You might also ask your doctor or nurse about **acupuncture**, which may help relieve nausea and vomiting caused by cancer treatment.

To learn more about dealing with nausea and vomiting during cancer treatment, see *Eating Hints: Before, During, and After Cancer Treatment*, a book from the National Cancer Institute. You can get a free copy at http://www.cancer.gov/publications or 1-800-4-CANCER (1-800-422-6237).

Sexual and Fertility Changes

What They Are

Radiation therapy sometimes causes sexual changes, which can include hormone changes and loss of interest in or ability to have sex. It can also affect fertility during and after radiation therapy. For a woman, this means that she might not be able to get pregnant and have a baby. For a man, this means that he might not be able to get a woman pregnant. Sexual and fertility changes differ for men and women.

Be sure to tell your doctor iF you are pregnant beFore you start radiation therapy.

Problems for women include:
- Pain or discomfort when having sex
- Vaginal itching, burning, dryness, or atrophy (when the muscles in the vagina become weak and the walls of the vagina become thin)
- **Vaginal stenosis**, when the vagina becomes less elastic, narrows, and gets shorter
- Symptoms of menopause for women not yet in menopause. These include hot flashes, vaginal dryness, and not having your period.
- Not being able to get pregnant after radiation therapy is over

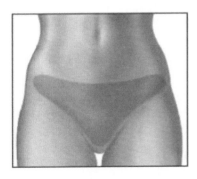

Radiation to the shaded area may cause sexual and fertility changes.

Problems for men include:

- **Impotence** (also called **erectile dysfunction** or ED), which means not being able to have or keep an erection
- Not being able to get a woman pregnant after radiation therapy is over due to fewer or less effective sperm

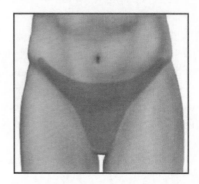

Why They Occur

Sexual and fertility changes can happen when people get radiation therapy to the pelvic area. For women, this includes radiation to the vagina, uterus, or ovaries. For men, this includes radiation to the testicles or prostate. Many sexual side effects are caused by scar tissue from radiation therapy. Other problems, such as fatigue, pain, anxiety, or depression, can affect your interest in having sex.

How Long They Last

After radiation therapy is over, most people want to have sex as much as they did before treatment. Many sexual side effects go away after treatment ends. But you may have problems with hormone changes and fertility for the rest of your life. If you are able to get pregnant or father a child after you have finished radiation therapy, it should not affect the health of the baby.

Ways to Manage

For both men and women, it is important to be open and honest with your spouse or partner about your feelings, concerns, and how you prefer to be intimate while you are getting radiation therapy.

For women, here are some issues to discuss with your doctor or nurse:

- **Fertility.** Before radiation therapy starts, let your doctor or nurse know if you think you might want to get pregnant after your treatment ends. He or she can talk with you about ways to preserve your fertility, such as preserving your eggs to use in the future.
- **Sexual problems.** You may or may not have sexual problems. Your doctor or nurse can tell you about side effects you can expect and suggest ways for coping with them.
- **Birth control.** It is very important that you do not get pregnant while having radiation therapy. Radiation therapy can hurt the fetus at all stages of pregnancy. If you have not yet gone through menopause, talk with your doctor or nurse about birth control and ways to keep from getting pregnant.
- **Pregnancy.** Make sure to tell your doctor or nurse if you are already pregnant.
- **Stretching your vagina.** Vaginal stenosis is a common problem for women who have radiation therapy to the pelvis. This can make it painful to have sex. You can help by stretching your vagina using a **dilator** (a device that gently stretches the tissues of the vagina). Ask your doctor or nurse where to find a dilator and how to use it.
- **Lubrication.** Use a special lotion for your vagina (such as Replens®) once a day to keep it moist. When you have sex, use a water- or mineral oil-based lubricant (such as K-Y Jelly® or Astroglide®).
- **Sex.** Ask your doctor or nurse whether it is okay for you to have sex during radiation therapy. Most women can have sex, but it is a good idea to ask and be sure. If sex is painful due to vaginal dryness, you can use a water- or mineral oil-based lubricant.

For men, here are some issues to discuss with your doctor or nurse:

- **Fertility.** Before you start radiation therapy, let your doctor or nurse know if you think you might want to father children in the future. He or she may talk with you about ways to preserve your fertility before treatment starts, such as banking your sperm. Your sperm will need to be collected before you begin radiation therapy.
- **Impotence.** Your doctor or nurse can let you know whether you are likely to become impotent and how long it might last. Your doctor can prescribe medicine or other treatments that may help.

- **Sex.** Ask if it is okay for you to have sex during radiation therapy. Most men can have sex, but it is a good idea to ask and be sure.

Ways to learn more American Cancer Society

Offers a variety of services to patients and their families. It also supports research, provides printed materials, and conducts educational programs.

Toll-free: 1-800-ACS-2345 (1-800-227-2345)

Phone: 404-320-3333

Online: http://www.cancer

fertileHope

Dedicated to helping people with cancer faced with infertility.

Toll-free: 1-888-994-HOPE (1-888-994-4673)

Online: http://www.fertilehope.org

Skin Changes

What They Are

Radiation therapy can cause skin changes in your treatment area. Here are some common skin changes:

- **Redness.** Your skin in the treatment area may look as if you have a mild to severe sunburn or tan. This can occur on any part of your body where you are getting radiation.
- **Pruritus.** The skin in your treatment area may itch so much that you always feel like scratching. This causes problems because scratching too much can lead to **skin breakdown** and infection.
- **Dry and peeling skin.** This is when the skin in your treatment area gets very dry— much drier than normal. In fact, your skin may be so dry that it peels like it does after a sunburn.
- **Moist reaction.** Radiation kills skin cells in your treatment area, causing your skin to peel off faster than it can grow back. When this happens, you can get sores or ulcers. The skin in your treatment area can also become wet, sore, or infected. This is more common where you have skin folds, such as your buttocks, behind your ears, under your breasts. It may also occur where your skin is very thin, such as your neck.
- **Swollen skin.** The skin in your treatment area may be swollen and puffy.

Why They Occur

Radiation therapy causes skin cells to break down and die. When people get radiation almost every day, their skin cells do not have enough time to grow back between treatments. Skin changes can happen on any part of the body that gets radiation.

How Long They Last

Skin changes may start a few weeks after you begin radiation therapy. Many of these changes often go away a few weeks after treatment is over. But even after radiation therapy ends, you may still have skin changes. Your treated skin may always look darker and blotchy. It may feel very dry or thicker than before. And you may always burn quickly and be sensitive to the sun. You will always be at risk for skin cancer in the treatment area. Be sure to avoid tanning beds and protect yourself from the sun by wearing a hat, long sleeves, long pants, and sunscreen with an SPF of 30 or higher.

Ways to Manage

- **Skin care.** Take extra good care of your skin during radiation therapy. Be gentle and do not rub, scrub, or scratch in the treatment area. Also, use creams that your doctor prescribes.
- **Do not put anything on your skin that is very hot or cold.** This means not using heating pads, ice packs, or other hot or cold items on the treatment area. It also means washing with lukewarm water.
- **Be gentle when you shower or take a bath.** You can take a lukewarm shower every day. If you prefer to take a lukewarm bath, do so only every other day and soak for less than 30 minutes. Whether you take a shower or bath, make sure to use a mild soap that does not have fragrance or deodorant in it. Dry yourself with a soft towel by patting, not rubbing, your skin. Be careful not to wash off the ink markings that you need for radiation therapy.
- **Use only those lotions and skin products that your doctor or nurse suggests.** If you are using a prescribed cream for a skin problem or acne, you must tell your doctor or nurse before you begin radiation treatment. Check with your doctor or nurse before using any of the following skin products:
  - Bubble bath
  - Cornstarch
  - Cream
  - Deodorant

- Hair removers
- Makeup
- Oil
- Ointment
- Perfume
- Powder
- Soap
- Sunscreen

- **Cool, humid places.** Your skin may feel much better when you are in cool, humid places. You can make rooms more humid by putting a bowl of water on the radiator or using a humidifier. If you use a humidifier, be sure to follow the directions about cleaning it to prevent bacteria.
- **Soft fabrics.** Wear clothes and use bed sheets that are soft, such as those made from cotton.
- **Do not wear clothes that are tight and do not breathe,** such as girdles and pantyhose.
- **Protect your skin from the sun every day.** The sun can burn you even on cloudy days or when you are outside for just a few minutes. Do not go to the beach or sun bathe. Wear a broad-brimmed hat, long-sleeved shirt, and long pants when you are outside. Talk with your doctor or nurse about sunscreen lotions. He or she may suggest that you use a sunscreen with an SPF of 30 or higher. You will need to protect your skin from the sun even after radiation therapy is over, since you will have an increased risk of skin cancer for the rest of your life.
- **Do not use tanning beds.** Tanning beds expose you to the same harmful effects as the sun.
- **Adhesive tape.** Do not put bandages, BAND-AIDS®, or other types of sticky tape on your skin in the treatment area. Talk with your doctor or nurse about ways to bandage without tape.
- **Shaving.** Ask your doctor or nurse if you can shave the treated area. If you can shave, use an electric razor and do not use pre-shave lotion.
- **Rectal area.** If you have radiation therapy to the rectal area, you are likely to have skin problems. These problems are often worse after a bowel movement. Clean yourself with a baby wipe or squirt of water from a spray bottle. Also ask your nurse about sitz baths (a warm-

water bath taken in a sitting position that covers only the hips and buttocks.)

- **Talk with your doctor or nurse.** Some skin changes can be very serious. Your treatment team will check for skin changes each time you have radiation therapy. Make sure to report any skin changes that you notice.
- **Medicine.** Medicines can help with some skin changes. They include lotions for dry or itchy skin, antibiotics to treat infection, and other drugs to reduce swelling or itching.

Throat Changes

What They Are
Radiation therapy to the neck or chest can cause the lining of your throat to become inflamed and sore. This is called **esophagitis**. You may feel as if you have a lump in your throat or burning in your chest or throat. You may also have trouble swallowing.

Why They Occur
Radiation therapy to the neck or chest can cause throat changes because it not only kills cancer cells, but can also damage the healthy cells that line your throat. Your risk for throat changes depends on how much radiation you are getting, whether you are also having chemotherapy, and whether you use tobacco and alcohol while you are getting radiation therapy.

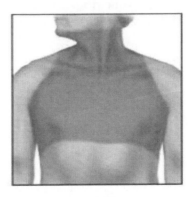

Radiation to the shaded area may cause throat changes.

How Long They Last

You may notice throat changes 2 to 3 weeks after starting radiation. You will most likely feel better 4 to 6 weeks after radiation therapy has finished.

Ways to Manage

- **Be careful what you eat when your throat is sore.**
  - Choose foods that are easy to swallow.
  - Cut, blend, or shred foods to make them easier to eat.
  - Eat moist, soft foods such as cooked cereals, mashed potatoes, and scrambled eggs.
  - Wet and soften food with gravy, sauce, broth, yogurt, or other liquids.
  - Drink cool drinks.
  - Sip drinks through a straw.
  - Eat foods that are cool or at room temperature.
- **Eat small meals and snacks.** It may be easier to eat a small amount of food at one time. Instead of eating 3 large meals each day, you may want to eat 5 or 6 small meals and snacks.
- **Choose foods and drinks that are high in calories and protein.** When it hurts to swallow, you may eat less and lose weight. It is important to keep your weight the same during radiation therapy. Having foods and drinks that are high in calories and protein can help you. See the chart of foods and drinks that are high in calories and protein later in this chapter.
- **Sit upright and bend your head slightly forward when you are eating or drinking.** Remain sitting or standing upright for at least 30 minutes after eating.
- **Don't have things that can burn or scrape your throat, such as:**
  - Hot foods and drinks
  - Spicy foods
  - Foods and juices that are high in acid, such as tomatoes and oranges
  - Sharp, crunchy foods such as potato or corn chips
  - All tobacco products, such as cigarettes, pipes, cigars, and chewing tobacco
  - Drinks that contain alcohol
- **Talk with a dietitian.** He or she can help make sure you eat enough to maintain your weight. This may include choosing foods that are high in calories and protein and foods that are easy to swallow.

- **Talk with your doctor or nurse.** Let your doctor or nurse know if you notice throat changes, such as trouble swallowing, feeling as if you are choking, or coughing while eating or drinking. Also, let him or her know if you have pain or lose any weight. Your doctor can prescribe medicines that may help relieve your symptoms, such as antacids, gels that coat your throat, and pain killers.

Ways to Learn More

To learn more about dealing with throat problems, the following books from the National Cancer Institute may help you: *Eating Hints: Before, During, and After Cancer Treatment* and *Pain Control: Support for People With Cancer*. You can get free copies at www.cancer or by calling 1-800-4-CANCER (1-800-422-6237).

Smokefree.gov

Provides resources, including information on quit lines, a step-by-step cessation guide, and publications, to help you or someone you care about quit smoking.

Toll-free: 1-877-44U-QUIT (1-877-448-7848)

Online: http://www.smokefree.gov

Urinary and Bladder Changes

What They Are

Radiation therapy can cause urinary and bladder problems, which can include:

- Burning or pain when you begin to **urinate** or after you empty your bladder
- Trouble starting to urinate
- Trouble emptying your bladder
- Frequent, urgent need to urinate
- **Cystitis**, a swelling (**inflammation**) in your urinary tract
- **Incontinence**, when you cannot control the flow of urine from your bladder, especially when coughing or sneezing
- Frequent need to get up during sleep to urinate
- Blood in your urine
- Bladder spasms, which are like painful muscle cramps

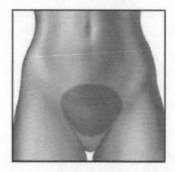

Radiation to the shaded area may cause urinary and bladder changes.

Why They Occur

Urinary and bladder problems may occur when people get radiation therapy to the prostate or bladder. Radiation therapy can harm the healthy cells of the bladder wall and urinary tract, which can cause inflammation, ulcers, and infection.

How Long They Last

Urinary and bladder problems often start 3 to 5 weeks after radiation therapy begins. Most problems go away 2 to 8 weeks after treatment is over.

Ways to Manage

- **Drink a lot of fluids.** This means 6 to 8 cups of fluids each day. Drink enough fluids so that your urine is clear to light yellow in color.
- **Avoid coffee, black tea, alcohol, spices, and all tobacco products.**
- **Talk with your doctor or nurse if you think you have urinary or bladder problems.** He or she may ask for a urine sample to make sure that you do not have an infection.
- **Talk to your doctor or nurse if you have incontinence.** He or she may refer you to a physical therapist who will assess your problem. The therapist can give you exercises to improve bladder control.
- **Medicine.** Your doctor may prescribe antibiotics if your problems are caused by an infection. Other medicines can help you urinate, reduce burning or pain, and ease bladder spasms.

Late Side Effects

Late side effects are those that first occur at least 6 months after radiation therapy is over. Late side effects are rare, but they do happen. It is important to have follow-up care with a radiation oncologist or nurse practitioner for the rest of your life.

Whether you get late side effects will depend on:

- The part of your body that was treated
- The dose and length of your radiation therapy
- If you received chemotherapy before, during, or after radiation therapy

Your doctor or nurse will talk with you about late side effects and discuss ways to help prevent them, symptoms to look for, and how to treat them if they occur.

Some late side effects are brain problems, infertility, joint problems, **lymphedema**, mouth problems, and secondary cancers.

Brain Changes

What They Are

Radiation therapy to the brain can cause problems months or years after treatment ends. Side effects can include memory loss, problems doing math, movement problems, incontinence, trouble thinking, or personality changes. Sometimes, dead tumor cells can form a mass in the brain, which is called radiation necrosis.

Ways to Manage

You will need to have check-ups with your doctor or nurse for the rest of your life. If you have symptoms, you will have tests to see whether they are due to the cancer or late side effects.

If you have late side effects, your doctor or nurse practitioner:

- Will talk with you about ways to manage late side effects
- May refer you to a physical, occupational, or speech therapist who can help with problems caused by late side effects
- May prescribe medicine or suggest surgery to help with the symptoms

Infertility

What it is

For men, infertility means not being able to get a woman pregnant. For women, it means not being able to get pregnant.

Ways men with infertility can become a parent:

- **Donor sperm.** This means getting a woman pregnant with sperm given by another man.
- **Adoption.** Taking on legal responsibility for someone else's child and raising the child as your own.

Ways women with infertility can become a parent:

- **Donor embryos.** Another couple donates a fertilized egg that your doctor implants in your uterus to carry until birth.
- **Donor eggs.** An egg (donated by someone else) is fertilized by your partner's sperm. Your doctor implants the fertilized egg in your uterus to carry until birth.
- **Surrogacy.** Another woman carries and gives birth to your child. She can also donate her egg, which is fertilized by your partner's sperm.
- **Adoption.** Taking on legal responsibility for someone else's child and raising the child as your own.

Joint Changes

What They Are

Radiation therapy can cause scar tissue and weakness in the part of the body that was treated. This can lead to loss of motion in your joints, such as your jaw, shoulders, or hips. Joint problems can show up months or years after radiation therapy is over.

Ways to Manage

Notice early signs of joint problems. These signs include:

- Trouble getting your mouth to open wide
- Pain when you make certain movements, such as reaching over your head or putting your hand in a back pocket

Talk with your doctor or nurse. He or she may refer you to a physical therapist who will assess your joint problems. The therapist can give you exercises to decrease pain, increase strength, and improve movement.

Lymphedema

What It Is

Swelling in an arm or a leg caused by a build up of lymph fluid. Lymphedema can happen if your lymph nodes were removed during surgery or damaged by radiation therapy.

Tell your doctor or nurse if you notice swelling in the arm or leg on the side where you had radiation.

Ways to Manage

- **Meet with your doctor or nurse.** Ask about your risk of lymphedema and ways to prevent it. Your doctor or nurse may suggest exercises, medicines, or compression garments (special wraps to put on your legs or arms). You might also want to ask for a referral to a physical therapist.
- **Be active**. Exercise can help prevent and treat lymphedema. Ask your doctor, nurse, or physical therapist which exercises are safe for you to do.
- **Take care of your arm or leg.**
    - Use skin lotion at least once a day.
    - Avoid sunburn. Use sunscreen with an SPF of 30 or higher and wear long sleeves and long pants if you need to be in the sun.
    - Wear gloves when you garden or cook.
    - Clip your toenails straight across, file your fingernails, and do not cut your cuticles.
    - Keep your feet clean and wear dry, cotton socks.
    - Clean cuts with soap and water and then use antibacterial ointment.
    - Avoid extreme hot or cold, such as ice packs or heating pads.
    - Do not put pressure on your arm or leg. For example, do not cross your legs when sitting or carry your purse on the side that had radiation.
    - Wear loose clothes that do not have tight elastic cuffs or waistbands.

- **Notice early signs of lymphedema.** Let your doctor or nurse know if you have:
- Pain or a sense of heaviness in your arm or leg
- A feeling of tightness in your arm or leg
- Trouble putting on your shoes or rings
- Weakness in your arm or leg
- Redness, swelling, or other signs of infection

Mouth Changes

What They Are

Radiation therapy to your head and neck can cause late side effects in your mouth. Problems may include dry mouth, cavities, or bone loss in the jaw.

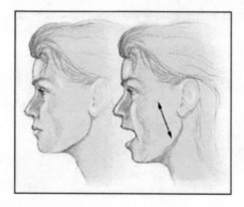

Exercise your jaw 3 times a day.

Ways to Manage

- **Visit your dentist.** You may be asked to have your teeth checked every 1 to 2 months for at least 6 months after radiation treatment ends. During this time, your dentist will look for changes in your mouth, teeth, and jaw.
- **Exercise your jaw.** Open and close your mouth 20 times as far as you can without causing pain. Do this exercise 3 times a day, even if your jaw isn't stiff.
- **Take good care of your teeth and gums.** This means flossing, using daily fluoride treatments, and brushing your teeth after meals and before you go to bed.

- **Have your dentist contact your radiation oncologist before you have dental or gum surgery.** This includes not having teeth pulled from the part of your mouth that received radiation. There may be other options than surgery.

Secondary Cancer

What It Is
Radiation therapy can cause a new cancer many years after you have finished treatment. This does not happen very often.

Ways to Manage
You will need to have check-ups with your radiation oncologist or nurse practitioner for the rest of your life to check for cancer—the one you were treated for and any new cancer that may occur.

See Resources for Learning More later in this chapter for ways to learn more about late side effects.

QUESTIONS TO ASK YOUR DOCTOR OR NURSE

What kind of radiation therapy will I get?

How can radiation therapy help?

How many weeks will my course of radiation therapy last?

What kinds of side effects should I expect during my course of radiation therapy?

Will these side effects go away after radiation therapy is over?

What kind of late side effects should I expect after radiation therapy is over?

What can I do to manage these side effects?

What will you do to manage these side effects?

How can I learn more about radiation therapy?

LISTS OF FOODS AND LIQUIDS

Clear Liquids

This list may help if you have diarrhea.

Types of Liquids	Includes . . .
Soups	Bouillon Clear, fat-free broth Consommé Strained vegetable broth
Drinks	Apple juice Clear carbonated beverages Cranberry or grape juice Fruit-flavored drinks Fruit punch Sports drinks Tea Water

Types of Liquids	Includes . . .
Sweets	Fruit ices without fruit pieces Fruit ices without milk Honey Jelly Plain gelatin dessert Popsicles

Foods and Drinks That Are High in Calories or Protein

This list may help if you need ideas for keeping your weight the same.

Types of Foods and Drinks	Includes . . .
Soups	Cream soups
Drinks	Instant breakfast shakes Milkshakes Whole milk (instead of low-fat or skim)
Main meals and other foods	Beans, legumes Butter, margarine, or oil Cheese Chicken, fish, or beef Cottage cheese Cream cheese on crackers or celery Deviled ham Eggs, such as scrambled or deviled eggs Muffins Nuts, seeds, wheat germ Peanut butter
Desserts and other sweets	Custards Frozen yogurt Ice cream Puddings Yogurt
Replacements and other supplements	Powdered milk added to foods (pudding, milkshakes, or scrambled eggs) High-protein supplements, such as Ensure® and Carnation® Instant Breakfast®

Foods and Drinks That Are Easy on the Stomach

This list may help if you have diarrhea or nausea and vomiting.

Types of Foods and Drinks	Includes . . .
Soups	Clear broth, such as chicken or beef
Drinks	Clear carbonated beverages Cranberry or grape juice Fruit-flavored drinks Fruit punch Sports drinks Tea Water
Main meals and snacks	Boiled potatoes Chicken, broiled or baked without the skin Crackers Cream of wheat Noodles Oatmeal Pretzels Rice Toast
Sweets	Angel food cake Canned peaches Gelatin Sherbet Yogurt

WORDS TO KNOW

3-D conformal radiation therapy (ray-dee-AY-shun): Uses a computer to create a 3-D picture of a cancer tumor. This allows doctors to give the highest possible dose of radiation to the tumor, while sparing the normal tissue as much as possible.

Acupuncture (AK-yoo-PUNK-cher): A technique of inserting thin needles through the skin at specific points on the body to control pain and side effects. It is a type of complementary and alternative medicine.

Alopecia (al-oh-PEE-shuh): Hair loss; when some or all of your hair falls out.

Anemia (a-NEE-mee-a): A problem in which the number of red blood cells is below normal.

Applicator: A large device used to place brachytherapy in the body.

Brachytherapy (BRAKE-ee-THER-a-pee): Treatment in which a solid radioactive substance is implanted inside your body, near or next to the cancer cells.

CT scan: A series of detailed pictures of areas inside the body, taken from different angles; the pictures are created by a computer linked to an x-ray machine.

Catheter: A flexible tube used to place brachytherapy in the body.

Course of treatment: All of your radiation therapy sessions.

Cystitis: Inflammation in your urinary tract.

Diet: Foods you eat (does not always refer to a way to lose weight).

Dilator (DYE-lay-tor): A device that gently stretches the tissues of the vagina.

Dry heaves: A problem that occurs when your body tries to vomit even though your stomach is empty.

Erectile dysfunction (e-WRECK-tile dis-FUNK-shun): Not able to have an erection of the penis adequate for sexual intercourse. Also called impotence.

Esophagitis: Inflammation of the esophagus (the tube that carries food from the mouth to the stomach).

External beam radiation therapy (ray-dee-AY-shun): Treatment in which a radiation source from outside your body aims radiation at your cancer cells.

Fatigue: A feeling of being weary or exhausted.

Follow-up care: Check-up appointments that you have after your course of radiation therapy is over.

Hyperfractionated radiation therapy ((hy-per-FRAK-shuh-NAYT-id ray-dee-AY-shun THAYR-uh-pee): Treatment in which radiation is given in smaller doses twice a day.

Imaging tests: Tests that produce pictures of areas inside the body.

Implant: Radioactive material put in your body through a sealed thin wire, catheter, or tube.

Impotence (IM-po-tense): Not able to have an erection of the penis adequate for sexual intercourse. Also called erectile dysfunction.

IMRT (intensity-modulated radiation therapy): A technique that uses a computer to deliver precise radiation doses to a cancer tumor or specific areas within the tumor.

Incontinence (in-KAHN-tih-nens): A problem in which you cannot control the flow of urine from your bladder.

Infertility: Not being able to produce children.

Inflammation: Redness, swelling, pain, and/or a feeling of heat in an area of the body.

Internal radiation therapy (ray-dee-AY-shun): Treatment in which a radioactive substance is put inside your body.

Intraoperative radiation (ray-dee-AY-shun): Radiation treatment aimed directly at cancer during surgery.

Late side effects: Side effects that first occur 6 or more months after radiation therapy is finished.

Local treatment: Radiation is aimed at only the part of your body with cancer.

Lymphedema: A problem in which excess fluid collects in tissue and causes swelling. It may occur in the arm or leg after lymph vessels or lymph nodes in the underarm or groin are removed by surgery or treated with radiation.

Medical leave: Taking time off work for a while due to a medical problem.

MRI (magnetic resonance imaging): A procedure in which radio waves and a powerful magnet linked to a computer are used to create detailed pictures of areas inside the body.

Nausea: When you have an upset stomach or queasy feeling and feel like you are going to throw up.

Pelvis: The area between your legs. Also called the groin.

Permanent implants: Radioactive pellets or seeds that always stay in your body.

PET (Positron emission tomography) scan: A procedure in which a small amount of radioactive glucose (sugar) is injected into a vein, and a scanner is used to make detailed, computerized pictures of areas inside the body where the glucose is used. Because cancer cells often use more glucose than normal cells, the pictures can be used to find cancer cells in the body.

Pruritus: Severe itching.

Psychostimulants: Medicines that can help decrease fatigue, give a sense of well-being, and increase appetite.

Radiation necrosis: A problem in which dead tumor cells form a mass in the brain.

Radiation oncologist (ray-dee-AY-shun on-KO-lo-jist): A doctor who specializes in using radiation to treat cancer.

Radiation therapy (ray-dee-AY-shun): High doses of radiation used to treat cancer and other diseases.

Radiotherapy (RAY-dee-o-THER-a-pee): Another word for radiation therapy.

Simulation (sim-you-LAY-shun): A process used to plan radiation therapy so that the target area is precisely located and marked.

Sitz bath: A warm-water bath taken in a sitting position that covers only the hips and buttocks.

Skin breakdown: A side effect from radiation therapy in which the skin in the treatment area peels off faster than it can grow back.

Support groups: Meetings for people who share the same problems, such as cancer.

Treatment field: One or more places on your body where the radiation will be aimed. Also called treatment port.

Treatment port: One or more places on your body where the radiation will be aimed. Also called treatment field.

Urinate (YOOR-in-nate): Emptying your bladder of urine.

Vaginal stenosis (ste-NO-sis): A problem in which the vagina narrows and gets smaller. **Vomiting**: When you get sick and throw up your food.

Xerostomia: Dry mouth.

RESOURCES FOR LEARNING MORE

National Cancer Institute Cancer Information Service
Answers questions about cancer clinical trials and cancer-related services and helps users find information on the NCI Web site. Provides NCI printed materials.

Toll-free: 1-800-4-CANCER (1-800-422-6237)
TTY: 1-800-332-8615
Online: http://www.cancer
Chat online: http://www.cancer

American Cancer Society
Offers a variety of services to patients and their families. It also supports research, provides printed materials, and conducts educational programs.

Toll-free: 1-800-ACS-2345 (1-800-227-2345)
Online: http://www.cancer

American Society for Therapeutic Radiology and Oncology
A society of radiation oncology professionals who specialize in treating patients with radiation therapy. Patients can get information on treating cancer with radiation and find a radiation oncologist in their area.

Toll-free: 1-800-962-7876
Online: http://www.astro.org

CancerCare, Inc.
Offers free support, information, financial assistance, and practical help to people with cancer and their loved ones.
Toll-free: 1-800-813-HOPE (1-800-813-4673)
Online: http://www.cancercare.org
E-mail: info@cancercare.org

fertileHOPE
Dedicated to helping people with cancer faced with infertility.
Toll-free: 1-888-994-HOPE (1-888-994-4673)
Online: http://www.fertilehope.org

National Brain Tumor Foundation
Dedicated to providing information and support for brain tumor patients, their family members, and health care professionals, while supporting innovative research into better treatment options and a cure for brain tumors.
Toll-free: 1-800-934-2873
Online: http://www.braintumor.org

National Lymphedema Network
Provides education and guidance to lymphedema patients, health care professionals, and the general public by disseminating information on the prevention and management of primary and secondary lymphedema.
Toll-free: 800-541-3259
Phone: 510-208-3200
Online: http://www.lymphnet.org
E-mail: nln@lymphnet.org

National Oral Health Information Clearinghouse
A service of the National Institute of Dental and Craniofacial Research that provides oral health information for special care patients.
Phone: 301-402-7364
Online: http://www.nidcr.nih.gov

The Wellness Community
Provides free psychological and emotional support to cancer patients and their loved ones.

Toll-free: 1-888-793-WELL (1-888-793-9355)
Phone: 202-659-9709
Online: http://www.thewellnesscommunity.org
E-mail: help@thewellnesscommunity.org

INDEX

D

E

F

training, 59
transfusion, 18
trial, 9
tumor(s), 3, 52, 57, 95, 102, 103, 104, 106
tumor cells, 95, 104

U

urinary tract, 93, 94, 103
urine, 18, 28, 42, 51, 68, 93, 94, 103, 105
uterus, 66, 86, 96

V

vaccine, 26, 27
vagina, 38, 85, 86, 87, 103, 105
vegetables, 20, 21, 27, 47, 75
vein, 5, 104
vessels, 104
vision, 19, 44, 73
visualization, 22
vitamins, 7, 15, 16, 17, 18
vomiting, 13, 14, 32, 33, 34, 48, 50, 51, 62,
    72, 83, 84, 85, 101

W

walking, 11, 19, 35, 39, 70
waste, 27
water, 17, 19, 20, 21, 22, 26, 27, 31, 35, 38,
    41, 44, 70, 75, 81, 87, 89, 90, 97, 105
weakness, 16, 34, 96
wear, 31, 35, 38, 44, 64, 81, 90, 97
weight gain, 16
weight loss, 16
well-being, 23, 77, 104
wheat germ, 46, 101
wheezing, 41
white blood cell count, 26
white blood cells, 25, 26, 51
worry, 12, 62, 70
wrists, 18

X

xerostomia, 80
x-rays, vii, 7, 56, 61, 63, 65

Z

zinc, 41
zinc oxide, 41